£7.95

The Sexual Politics of Reproduction

The Sexual Politics of Reproduction

Edited by
Hilary Homans

Gower

Published by

Gower Publishing Company Limited
Gower House, Croft Road
Aldershot, Hants GU11 3HR, England

Gower Publishing Company
Old Post Road
Brookfield
Vermont 05036, USA

British Library Cataloguing in Publication Data

The sexual politics of reproduction
1. Human reproduction – Social aspects
I. Homans, Hilary
306.7 QP251

Library of Congress Cataloging in Publication Data

The sexual politics of reproduction
Bibliography: p.
Includes index.
1. Human reproduction – social aspects – addresses, essays, lectures. 2. Sex preselection – social aspects – addresses, essays, lectures.
I. Homans, Hilary. 1950–
HQ751.S5 1985 304.6'32 85-5625

ISBN 0-566-00853-X
0-566-05054-4 (Pbk)

Contents

	Acknowledgements	vi
	Notes on Contributors	vii
1	Introduction *Hilary Homans*	1
2	Male Power and Menstrual Etiquette *Sophie Laws*	13
3	The Hidden Pathology of the Male Reproductive System *Naomi Pfeffer*	30
4	The Medical Construction of the Contraceptive Career *Hilary Thomas*	45
5	Sex and the Contraceptive Act *Scarlet Pollock*	64
6	Legal Abortion in Great Britain *Madeleine Simms*	78
7	Who's for Amniocentesis? The Politics of Prenatal Screening *Wendy Farrant*	96
8	By Design: Reproductive Strategies and the Meaning of Motherhood *Ellen Lewin*	123
9	Discomforts in Pregnancy: Traditional Remedies and Medical Prescriptions *Hilary Homans*	139
	Bibliography	163
	List of Useful Addresses	178
	Name Index	181
	Subject Index	186

Acknowledgements

Thanks are due to each of the contributors for making this book possible, and to the British Sociological Association (BSA) Human Reproduction Study Group for providing a forum for presenting papers and lively debate. Sheila Roche (former convenor of the group) and Jo Garcia (present convenor) deserve special thanks in this respect.

Lorna McKee provided much useful information about the practicalities of publishing, and Caroline Lane has encouraged the book along the way. Mike Milotte of the BSA should be thanked for undertaking to sponsor the book. Typing of various drafts has been carried out by Norma Bainbridge, Ruth Elkan, Dorothy Foster and Jeanette Whitmore.

Intellectual encouragement has been received from the feminist research group of Warwick/Leamington, in particular Loraine Blaxter, Celia Davies and Sophie Laws; and practical help from Deborah Gerrard and Caroline Sheldrick.

Finally, thanks to Celia Davies and Antoinette Satow for providing tremendous sisterly support in the final stages of the book, and to my son Mark for giving practical help and being his usual cheerful self.

Contributors

Wendy Farrant is a member of the Women's Health Information Centre (WHIC) collective. Her interest in the politics of health originates from living in East Africa and teaching medical students at the University of Dar-es-Salaam in the early 1970s. Since returning to Britain she has pursued that interest through involvement in the Politics of Health Group (POHG), WHIC, her local Community Health Council and research into women's health and health education.

Hilary Homans is actively involved in the women's health movement and is a member of the London-based Women's Health Information Centre (WHIC) collective. She has been involved for the past eight years in research into aspects of women's health, health education and women as health workers, and has taught women's health courses for many years. Together with Sheila Roche she jointly convened the British Sociological Association Human Reproduction Study Group from 1980 to 1982.

Sophie Laws is actively involved in the Women's Liberation movement. The paper published in this volume is drawn from work she is doing as a postgraduate student at Warwick University on the social meanings of menstruation. She is a member of the editorial collective of the radical feminist magazine *Trouble and Strife*.

Ellen Lewin After receiving her doctorate in Anthropology from Stanford University in 1975, she taught at the University of California, San Francisco. Her research has focused on issues in the anthropology of gender and has included work with Latina immigrants, nurses, and single mothers. She is currently completing a book on single motherhood in America and is the co-editor, with Virginia Olesen, of *Women, Health and Healing: toward a new perspective*. She lives in San Francisco.

Naomi Pfeffer is co-author (with Anne Woollett) of *The Experience of Infertility* (Virago, 1983) and is currently researching twentieth century history of reproductive medicine.

Scarlet Pollock lives with a bad tempered house cow and her six calves, twelve hungry hens, a fat mare and her foal, too many chicks, ten warm cats, a thieving puppy, eleven ducklings and the same old lover. She enjoys almost every minute of it. She is co-editor (as Friedman) with Elisabeth Sarah of *On the Problem of Men* (The Women's Press, 1982); author of *Women, Sexuality and Contraception* (Routledge and Kegan Paul, forthcoming); and co-editor with Jo Sutton of *The Politics of Fatherhood* (The Women's Press, forthcoming).

Madeleine Simms is a medical sociologist and author of several studies on the historical and social aspects of the abortion law reform movement. She was formerly general secretary of the Abortion Law Reform Association and chairperson of the Co-ordinating Committee in Defence of the 1967 Abortion Act.

Hilary Thomas is a medical sociology Research Fellow at Hughes Hall, Cambridge, where she has been working with the Early Parenthood Project on the evaluation of a community antenatal clinic. She is writing a PhD thesis on women and contraception.

1 Introduction
Hilary Homans

Most of the papers in this collection have grown out of meetings of the British Sociological Association (BSA) Human Reproduction Study Group. This group which has been meeting now on a twice yearly basis for more than a decade, started with a relatively narrow view of the sociological study of reproduction among humans and focused much of its attention on contraception, pregnancy and motherhood. Its registers of research into the sociology of Human Reproduction reflect this (Scambler and Versluysen, 1976; Oakley, 1976a and Macintyre, 1978). The narrow way in which human reproduction was defined in the early days of the group was made explicit by Oakley:

> 'Reproduction' is interpreted as 'the action or process of forming, creating, or bringing into existence again' (Oxford English Dictionary). Thus actions or processes relating to conception, pregnancy, birth and lactation are included. The following topics, which could be considered thematically connected to reproduction have been omitted: human sexuality and sexual behaviour; the study of sexually transmitted diseases; social factors in, or the epidemiology of other diseases of the reproductive organs; infant care and infant feeding . . . . (1976a: Introduction, *Bibliography on the Sociology of Human Reproduction*).

Over the years, however, this limited definition of the sociology of human reproduction within the study group has broadened to encompass the study of sexuality, reproductive pathologies, reproductive technology and the social relations governing reproductive processes. During the years 1980 to 1982, when Sheila Roche and I jointly convened the Human Reproduction Study Group, we were as feminists concerned to look at the politics of reproduction and the meetings of the group during this period were organised around this theme.

This collection then presents work which explores the political forces involved in reproductive processes. Some contributors look explicitly at sexual politics and the maintenance of patriarchal social relations (Laws and Pollock). Others look at the construction of medical knowledge and what this means for our understanding of male reproductive systems (Pfeffer), contraceptive choice (Thomas), or health care in pregnancy (Homans). The political forces which led to the legalisation of abortion in Britain are described in detail by Madeleine Simms, while Wendy Farrant examines closely the vested interests and resulting contradictions present in prenatal screening programmes. Ellen Lewin's contribution, the only one which was not originally presented at a meeting of the Human Reproduction Study Group,[1] shows how women actively seek out motherhood through artificial insemination and achieve this either by using medical services, or their own networks and resources.

All of the chapters attempt to get away from definitions of reproductive processes as biological events isolated from social reality. At the same time the authors are wary of a social constructionist approach which, through stressing social aspects, masks the effect of biology on our lives (for a critique, cf Sayers, 1982, p. 124; Riley, 1983). We are all aware that menstruation and childbirth can be painful events and recognise the problems that heterosexual women may have in preventing pregnancy or obtaining an abortion. We are also aware of the difficulties some women experience in attempting to become pregnant either because of infertility (Pfeffer and Woollett, 1983), or because they want to control the process themselves (Duelli Klein, 1984). However, we do not see biology as destiny, rather we see that the way services are organised, reproductive technologies controlled and our sexuality constrained, as being particular manifestations of male control over women which shapes our reproductive experiences.

The following sections locate the papers in this collection in the context of other literature on human reproduction. The papers address different aspects of the sexual politics of reproduction and ask questions about who controls reproduction; how is our knowledge about reproduction dominated by male views about women and what role does the medical profession play in all this; how is access to services tempered by the state and professional control; and in whose interests are technological developments. Reading these accounts we become aware of how complex the struggle for reproductive freedom is, and how decisions about our bodies are not individual matters, but political issues.

Male control and reproduction

Male control over reproduction is maintained at an individual level by the power men have over women, and at an institutional level through cultural practices and patriarchal ideology which shapes the way that all institutions in our society are organised. For instance, within medicine, negative views of women's reproductive systems have led to the development of a medical specialty (gynaecology) to detect and treat pathology, whereas for male reproductive systems no such specialty exists (see Pfeffer, this collection).

It is widely recognised that in most societies men control some aspects of human reproduction. Anthropologists who have written about this tend to view male control as being expressed through cultural practices (rites, rituals and taboos) which have resulted from men's fears of women's reproductive powers (Edholm *et al.*, 1977; Lindenbaum, 1972; Faithorn, 1975, p. 130; Kitzinger, 1978, pp. 226–7; Okely, 1977, p. 68). These writings have usually focused on how men within certain cultures control the sexuality and fertility of their women. However, we must be careful about passing judgement on what happens in other cultures, particularly if it is based on the assumed 'normality' of our own. For this can lead to the 'pathologising' of black culture by white researchers, who do not critically examine their own culture (cf Carby, 1982). Sophie Laws (this collection) quite rightly says that there is something racist in the way that 'our' (i.e. white) men 'are never made the focus of attention'.

Black feminists are attempting to redress this imbalance and there are recent studies which show clearly how white men controlled black women's sexuality and reproductive freedom during slavery in America (Hooks, 1981; Davis, 1982). Bell Hooks (1981) details the horrors black women were subjected to, including rape, torture and murder, for not complying with white male wishes (p. 28). In addition to being sexually debased, black women were used as breeding stock to increase the number of slaves and were reprimanded for failing to breed (pp. 39–40), while white women were exalted, seen as pure, innocent and asexual (p. 31).

While this book is predominantly about white culture, it is important that we are aware of the way in which male control over reproduction may affect groups of women differentially. In this context it is important that more research is funded so that black women have the opportunity to reveal the structures which shape their lives and reproductive experiences. It is also important that white researchers do not claim that their research is universal when it only refers to white culture, or to render black people invisible by ignoring them in population samples. For example, Farrant, Homans and Lewin (this collection) draw on data from samples which include black and ethnic minority group women because these women were represented in the populations under study.

An understanding of the process by which male control over reproduction is maintained can only be developed by our challenge of existing assumptions. For instance, some radical feminists have re-examined conventional beliefs about women and argued that many practices (such as the seclusion of menstruating women or the experience of motherhood), can be positively valued if it is women themselves who are determining the conditions of the experience (cf Rich, 1977b).

Sophie Laws (this collection) looks at the way that the concept of taboo has been used in relation to menstruation and argues that this is not particularly helpful in furthering our understanding of how patriarchal relations operate on a day-to-day basis. She prefers to look at the way in which men use etiquette to express their power over women. She carefully examines male culture (that is, what men say to other men) by looking at it in relation to menstrual etiquette. This approach is very important as we have very little information about male culture, particularly as it relates to reproduction. Many of the earlier feminist analyses concentrated on women's experiences, making women visible and giving them a voice through feminist writings.

While it is important to examine male and female culture separately because men and women have very different consciousnesses in relation to reproduction (O'Brien, 1981, p. 21), it is also necessary to look at the way women and men negotiate relationships concerning reproduction. Scarlet Pollock (this collection) explores some assumptions concerning contemporary sexual relations. She argues that over the past few years changes in contraceptive technology have had far reaching implications on heterosexual relationships. For it is now assumed by men that women can control their fertility and therefore be constantly sexually available. Sexual relations (according to Pollock) can be defined as an all-important power struggle between women and men, with contraception becoming central to this struggle. This demonstrates the importance of looking at contraceptive practice in the context of sexual relations and how it is not sociologically meaningful to study them separately.

Using data collected from women university students, Scarlet Pollock shows that the contraceptive method actually used often depends on the male partner and what is seen least to interfere with his pleasure. Hilary Thomas (this collection) adds a further dimension to this by focusing solely on the 'public' view of the medical profession as expressed in medical journals. This data clearly shows how the medical profession perpetuates certain ideas about who should and should not have children.

Professional control

The way in which professional control has been exerted over human reproduction can be found by reading male 'official' accounts about women's bodies and reproductive systems. There is now a substantial amount of feminist literature which describes the way in which male doctors and scientists view women's reproductive organs (Ehrenreich,

1974; Weiss, 1975; Daly, 1978; Ehrenreich and English, 1978; Birke and Best, 1980; Rich, 1977b) and the way in which in the past sexual surgery has been used to control women (Ehrenreich and English, 1973; Barker-Benfield, 1976). Genital mutilation is still practised worldwide (Daly, 1978) and female sexual surgery (particularly in the form of hysterectomy) is on the increase (Daly, 1978, p. 238; Reitz, 1981, p. 170; Marieskind, 1980, p. 19), particularly for black and Third World women (Mass, 1976, and Davis, 1982). It appears that in the United States hysterectomies are seen as 'a simple solution for everything from backaches to contraception' (Larned, 1974, p. 36), and in South America as a form of involuntary sterilisation (Mass, 1976). In Britain a medical audit of hysterectomies in a District hospital found that 64 per cent of all operations were performed for 'excessive menstruation' (Grant and Hussein, 1984).[2] Often these operations are carried out without any consideration of the problems women may experience in coming to terms with a hysterectomy (Webb and Wilson-Barnett, 1983).

Whilst there is a considerable body of literature which shows how women's reproductive organs are described in pathological terms and the many atrocities performed on them in the name of science, we do not have any corresponding view of male reproductive organs. Naomi Pfeffer (this collection) shows that male reproductive systems do not have such a history of being described in negative terms. Male organs have been positively portrayed in medical writings and assumed to be 'structurally efficient' (Pfeffer). But is this so? Pfeffer argues that this portrayal is far from accurate, and shows that scientific thought does not always follow a rational logic, but succumbs to unsubstantiated statements about the unproblematic nature of male fertility and reproductive systems. Because the language used to conceptualise male and female systems has been used differentially by male scientists we do not 'know' what status our current understandings of the reproductive process should have. Many questions are as yet unasked and unanswered, but Pfeffer starts the analysis by asking some awkward questions.

Another contributor (Hilary Thomas) looks at medical writings on the subject of contraception. She finds that these authors do not restrict their comments to the scientific efficacy or suitability of different contraceptive methods, they also make assessments of social factors (such as 'illegitimacy' and 'fecklessness') which contraception is also seen as preventing. It is therefore possible to see how these medical writers construct a contraceptive 'career', which is based on their perceptions of women's contraceptive needs. The assumption that there is a normal path or 'career' which all women follow, inevitably means that some women experience difficulties in obtaining the contraceptive method of their choice (Doyal, 1979, p. 230; Pollock, 1984). The way in which women's views of 'normal reproduction' differ from those held by members of the medical profession is illustrated by Sally Macintyre, in her paper on single parenthood and she concludes by saying that 'the assumption that we know what "normal reproduction" is, or is perceived to be like, is perhaps untenable at this historical time' (1976, p. 170).

Assumptions about appropriate sexual behaviour have long been part of medical practice. In the past, members of the medical profession condoned male double standards by not informing women if their husbands had given them venereal disease (Pankhurst, 1913, p. 737). More recently, assumptions have been made about the location, timing and frequency of sex, in addition to the number and sex of partners. For instance, people visiting Family Planning clinics to obtain sheaths may find they are only given a specific number (it varies from clinic to clinic, but one is known to give 6 packets to last twelve weeks). There is therefore a very clear message about the assumed norm of frequency of intercourse.

In relation to pregnancy, we find that medical views about whether or not pregnancy constitutes a 'natural' or potentially 'pathological' process tend to influence the treatments prescribed for minor illness episodes (Homans, this collection). Elsewhere, Graham and Oakley (1981) show how women and obstetricians subscribe to different 'frames of reference' concerning the management of reproduction, while other writers (e.g. Stoller Shaw, 1974) look at the racist and sexist practices in contemporary obstetric care.

However, there is not a monolithic body of medical knowledge, nor do all doctors hold the same views. Hilary Homans (this collection) argues that there are differences in perspective between obstetricians and general practitioners (GPs) in the way they view antenatal care, and moreover there are differences between individual GPs as to whether or not they will prescribe drugs in pregnancy. Farrant and Simms (also this collection) clearly show that doctors are divided about the abortion issue. This often has more to do with the doctor's religion than being a member of the medical profession.

What we find in practice is that aspects of our reproduction (for instance, control over fertility and childbirth) are influenced (if not in some instances determined) by individual men, members of the medical profession, the doctrines of different religions and the state (in terms of what provisions are made available). In fact the state has a long history of involvement in reproductive matters.

The role of the state in reproduction

The activities of the state in Britain can be regarded as reproducing ideas about women and women's place in society which are often enshrined in legislation. The sphere of human reproduction is no exception, and topics such as population control and who should have children are frequent anxieties for government bodies.

Historically, we find that certain issues assume prominence at particular times, for instance, at the turn of the century when there were fears about the health of the nation, we find that state interventions into motherhood were introduced (Davin, 1978, p. 13). The interventions at this time concerned what the future generation of citizens should be like and the conditions under which they should be brought up (Lewis, 1980). State intervention in motherhood at this time provided a legitimate reason for the involvement of health care professionals in instructing women how to become 'good' mothers (Davin, 1978; Lewis, 1980).

Campaigners for birth control in the late 1910s and early 1920s came into direct conflict with organs of the state. For instance, authors of publications giving advice about birth control were charged under the obscenity laws (Rowbotham, 1974, p. 150). Birth control clinics were illegal on the grounds that contraception would lead to moral degeneration. It was not until 1930 (after considerable campaigning by ardent birth controllers) that the Minister of Health agreed that local authority clinics could provide contraceptive advice to married women on medical grounds. This, as Doyal says, reflected 'a limited acceptance by the state of the necessity to provide women with the means to control their own fertility' (1979, p. 174). The relationship between contraception, the medical profession and the state is dealt with succinctly by Aitken-Swan (1977).

Later in the 1940s, concern about the falling birth rate was expressed in the Beveridge Report. This report introduced the idea of *planned* reproduction in an attempt to reinforce married women's economic dependence on their husbands and to encourage motherhood as a natural and central part of marriage (Bland *et al.*,1978, p. 50). The Family Endowment Society (of which Beveridge was a member) actively campaigned for the introduction of maternity and family allowances as a financial incentive towards motherhood, though Macnicol (1980) argues that these benefits were finally introduced to preserve the economic status quo (p. 217).

The post war baby boom solved the problem of the falling birth rate and by the 1960s concerns began to be expressed about over-population. It was during this period, the so-called 'sexual revolution' of the sixties, that new contraceptive methods were developed and the state legislated in favour of abortion for women who fulfilled certain criteria. Madeleine Simms (this collection) describes the political activity that led up to the 1967 Abortion Act and the limitations of the Act in terms of women controlling their own fertility. This historical exposition is extremely useful as it provides an insight into the parliamentary decision-making process and the intricate web of forces which determine the fate of women wanting an abortion. She concludes that the decision about terminations is a political matter, involving state legislation, rather than being the concern of individual women who want to control their fertility. Additionally, as with most other state services, there are tremendous inequalities in provision based on geographical area, race and social class.

Inequalities in provision

Madeleine Simms (this collection) shows how although abortion is legal in Britain and should be available under the National Health Service (NHS), there are tremendous regional variations and in some areas provision is so poor that women tend to go to the charitable agencies (such as the British Pregnancy Advisory Service, Pregnancy Advisory Service, Marie Stopes Clinic). These regional inequalities are also commented on by other writers (Doyal, 1979, p. 233; Savage, 1982) and are seen to result from a general lack of funding for terminations under the NHS and in some cases from the religious beliefs of individual consultants. In relation to prenatal screening, Wendy Farrant (this collection) also comments on inequalities in service provision. She says that apart from a concentration of research in a few 'high risk' areas, prenatal screening provision 'bears little relation to need as measured by congenital abnormality statistics'.

In addition to the inequalities in service provision, there are also variations in the level of women's knowledge of services and their particular health care needs. Simms (this collection) comments on the fact that black and ethnic minority women are ten times more likely to die from abortions than women born in Britain (this latter group will also of course include black and ethnic minority women). The reason for this differential mortality rate is unclear and would appear to be an area warranting further research.

In other areas of contraception, evidence shows that black and ethnic minority group women are more likely to be using certain contraceptive methods. Christopher (1980) in her study of Haringey domiciliary family planning service found that Asian women were twice as likely to be using the coil (IUCD) than all other women, and West Indian women were one and a half times more likely to be sterilised (p. 243). Savage (1982), drawing on data from her case studies as a consultant obstetrician, shows that some Afro-Caribbean women in Britain have been sterilised without their full consent and often as a condition of having an abortion. In relation to Depo-Provera (the injectable contraceptive) Jill Rakusen (1981) says that there is 'evidence for the widespread belief that black and Asian women are being singled out in a racist way as prime targets for DP' (p. 81).

It is generally recognised that cultural and religious factors shape contraceptive use (Christopher, 1980, p. 243) and as we have seen above, women from ethnic minority groups do receive different contraceptive methods. Yet in the medical journals Hilary Thomas studied, the contraceptive needs of black and ethnic minority women are 'rarely mentioned'. Also in relation to reproductive technology it appears that black and ethnic minority women (together with working class women) receive the least information about procedures and are therefore not in a position to make informed decisions (see Farrant). In relation to drugs in pregnancy, Homans shows how Punjabi women often do not have the same information about side-effects as most white women.

Reproductive technology

Reproductive technology is an area in which the various parties interested in controlling one particular aspect of reproduction come together. There are the women (or couples) who anticipate the birth of a healthy baby, the medical profession, state involvement through legislation and funding, the medical supplies industry and the Church. The debate about reproductive technology raises fundamental questions about the pressures on women to have children and the meaning of children to people; who has children and in what social context; the implications of disability; and the desired sex of children.

The development of technological procedures in pregnancy is described by Rakusen and Davidson (1982b) and one of the consequences outlined by Day (1982) in her discussion of post-natal depression. In the contribution by Wendy Farrant in this collection, she describes some of the contradictions inherent in one aspect of reproductive technology, amniocentesis. She shows the inconsistencies between government measures to reduce foetal abnormality through prenatal screening, whilst opposing abortion on demand. Other aspects of reproductive technology (e.g. In Vitro Fertilisation (IVF) and Artificial Insemination by Donor (AID)) have recently been discussed by bodies of the state in the Warnock Committee Report (1984). The notable feature of the report describing the techniques at issue in the government inquiry into human fertilisation and human embryology, is that it is assumed that reproduction should always take place in the context of married, heterosexual relations (Warnock Committee of Inquiry, 1984). The belief that procreation is the rightful result of marriage is firmly entrenched in the government guidelines.

The separation of biological reproduction from women's bodies (Rowland, 1984, p. 359) to the hands of male scientists, further removes our control over what happens to our bodies. There are also implications for the kinds of babies which will be born. For example, should only 'perfect' babies be born, and what about the implications of sex predetermination in those countries where boy babies are preferred?

The dilemmas facing women who are diagnosed as carrying a less than 'perfect' baby are outlined by Farrant in her contribution. She shows how members of the medical profession do not seem to recognise the difficulty some women face in deciding to proceed with a termination after an 'affected' foetus has been diagnosed. There seems to be an implicit assumption in performing amniocentesis that if the foetus is 'affected' it should be aborted. What this means to people with disabilities has far reaching consequences (Saxton, 1984, pp. 301–2) and the decision to terminate is not made any easier for women in the absence of good amniocentesis counselling (Farrant; Finger, 1984, p. 288; Saxton, 1984, p. 301). The different groups who have a vested interest in prenatal screening technology are also described by Wendy Farrant. She shows how members of the medical profession are divided about the benefits to be gained from prenatal screening and the way in which some doctors have no qualms about recommending abortion in the case of an 'affected' foetus, but would strongly resist any attempt for women to have the right to choose an abortion on social grounds.

The possible risks associated with amniocentesis tend to be played down whilst the incidence of foetal abnormality in 'at risk' mothers is often overstated. Saxton (1984) says that 95 per cent of all amniocenteses performed indicate no abnormality and 'their only function consists of reassuring parents that their baby is fine' (p. 308). Whilst there is a need for reassurance during pregnancy this should be conducted in a proper manner with full information, rather than in the context of the negative reassurance philosophy of much routine antenatal care, i.e. 'they would tell me if there was something wrong' (Homans, 1982, p. 252).

Another worrying aspect of amniocentesis relates to sex predetermination (Hanmer, 1981; Rowland, 1984, p. 361), and the possibility of 'pre-natal femicide' (Hoskins and Holmes, 1984). Whilst in Britain women who have amniocentesis are given the option of knowing the sex of the child *in utero*, in other countries, notably India and China, the foetus may be aborted if it is the 'wrong' sex, i.e. female. Chacko (1982) commenting on the situation in India, says that amniocentesis followed by selective abortion is a frequent practice. Jeffery and Jeffery also argue in the Indian context that 'female foeticide could rapidly become common' (1983, p. 656). At the present time amniocentesis in India is only available at a few urban centres and at a price which limits its use (Jeffery and Jeffery, 1983, p. 657), yet despite this, in the first few years of existence, the Bhandari Clinic in Amritsar performed over five hundred sex determinations through amniocentesis at a cost of 500 rupees, about £33 sterling equivalent (Roggencamp, 1984, p. 267). In a society in which boy children are favoured, the consequences of sex predetermination through amniocentesis are very damaging to women.

The way in which the medical profession has attempted to retain control over women's bodies through reproductive technology can be clearly seen in the case of Artificial Insemination by Donor (AID). Underpinning this technology is the belief that babies should be born into heterosexual relationships. In 1978 a London GP refused AID to a lesbian woman because he did not agree with lesbian motherhood (*Evening News*, 1978). However, it is possible for lesbian women to receive AID through charitable agencies such as the British Pregnancy Advisory Service (BPAS) and the Pregnancy Advisory Service (PAS) at a cost of about £50 (Duelli Klein, 1984, p. 389). What is interesting about AID though, is that it really is not a 'technological' procedure, but something that women can do themselves. Ellen Lewin (this collection) shows through data from her study of single parenthood in the United States that there were a small number of lesbian women who used AID to achieve motherhood. However, the strategies used to achieve this end varied from seeking AID from the medical profession through to obtaining a semen sample from a known male and inseminating herself in a romantic setting. Lewin sees the use of AID by the women as part of a rational decision-making process which must be placed in the context of the meaning of children to women in a patriarchal society. The use of self-insemination by lesbians in Britain is seen as a *political* act and a means of women gaining control over reproduction (Duelli Klein, 1984). However, self-insemination is not only used by lesbian women and as Hornstein (1984) points out, there is a 'growing number of single, heterosexual women who are choosing donor insemination as a way of getting pregnant' (p. 376).

Whilst self-insemination does give us some control over reproduction we should be careful not to over-romanticise it. Some women have difficulty in obtaining semen from suitable donors at the fertile time in their cycle and of course, they may not conceive immediately. For some women it is important to find donors who are in sympathy with the aims and politics of self-insemination. To help in this, the feminist self-insemination group in London has produced guidelines to educate donors about the procedure and what is expected of them.

Other aspects of reproductive technology, such as in vitro fertilisation (IVF) and embryo transfer, remove conception from the women's body to the devices of male scientists. The implications of these technologies are discussed elsewhere (Rose and Hanmer, 1976 and various articles in Arditti, Duelli Klein and Minden, 1984), and will not be dealt with here, other than to say that even assuming these technologies are beneficial to women, there is no guarantee that women could have equal access to them for the reasons discussed earlier.

In drawing together the different elements which impinge on reproduction we develop a clear sense of the politics involved. While the weight of the different forces may make it difficult for us to imagine playing a more active role in controlling our reproductive experiences, there is clearly evidence from feminist writings that women are taking more control over their bodies (Phillips and Rakusen, 1979; Mackeith, 1978). Also as we see from two of the accounts in this collection, some women themselves have a detailed knowledge of maintaining and restoring health during pregnancy (Homans) and can be active in seeking their desired goal of motherhood without having a male partner (Lewin).

Feminists, through analysing patriarchal structures and writing about women's experiences, are therefore isolating those areas which need to be challenged and at the same time developing their own strategies. Two areas of work pose particular challenges for feminists involved in research. The first is to ensure that in their research and writing they do not produce values which are insensitive to the experiences of certain groups, such as black, working class, disabled or lesbian women. We need to listen to the criticism of groups such as these and take them into account in our work.

The second challenge is related to the first in so far as it involves asking questions not previously thought of, and working in areas previously unresearched. Naomi Pfeffer does this in her chapter which studies male reproductive systems, through looking at written material. Sophie Laws takes this analysis one stage further when she enters the realm of male culture, or 'spooking from the locker room' as Daly (1978) calls it. In this context we are warned that we will hear disturbing things and Laws' account of menstrual etiquette is full of unpleasant male comments about women's bodies. These are statements we are not supposed to hear and we should prepare ourselves for our response, whether it be anger or incredulity. Some of us would prefer to protect ourselves from hearing what men say about women in the company of other men, and perhaps are not ready or able to meet this challenge. Others, including some contributors to this volume, see it as important to face painful knowledge directly – to discover what we can learn from it and work out how changes can be made.

Notes

1. Ellen Lewin first presented her paper at the Society for Applied Anthropology conference, at Edinburgh in April, 1981.
2. I am grateful to Angela Coulter for drawing this research to my attention.

2 Male Power and Menstrual Etiquette

Sophie Laws

My project in this chapter is to sketch out a new kind of feminist analysis of the way in which menstruation is dealt with in British society. I have found that some of the terms used most frequently in discussion of social practices relating to menstruation tend to conceal more than they reveal. In relation to this culture, the idea that what we have is a 'menstrual taboo' which 'society' upholds, is oversimplified and in some ways misleading. Using data from interviews with men, I will describe the way in which men-only groups discuss menstruation, and will consider how this fits into the general pattern of men's power over women. Particularly we can see an etiquette of menstruation as part of a wider etiquette which governs the relations between women and men, marking and reinforcing each person's membership of one or other social group, and expressing their different statuses (Rich, 1977b, p. 57).

Social attitudes towards menstruation are usually discussed as a set of cultural ideas, or even as an ideology, which arrives within the culture almost from outside, from above or from the past – they are disembodied 'myths'. To give an example of this routine kind of logic, here is an extract from the section on 'Society's attitude' in Judy Lever's book on premenstrual tension:

> Society, since way back when, has generally treated menstruation as something to be ashamed of and hidden away, in contrast to pregnancy (the other side of menstruation) which is a proud event to be announced and welcomed. In many early primitive societies, women were, and in some tribes still are, banished from the main house and made to stay in a private hut during menstruation. They may not bathe, eat or touch their bodies, and have to remain in a crouched position the whole time. Above all, no men can come near them during this time, for fear of their lives. (Lever, 1979, p. 58)

She then goes on to list assorted European beliefs about menstruation, mentions the curse of Eve and then on to Greek Orthodox, Hindu and Orthodox Jewish rules relating to menstruation. These are taken as somehow explanatory of 'our' society's ways, which are not clearly spelt out.

This approach seems to be particularly inappropriate to the phenomenon it seeks to account for, because one of the striking things concerning ideas about menstruation within our culture, is that they conflict with one another and are often inconsistent. It is not possible to produce a clear account of 'what we think' about it for this reason.

Further, I see people as active creators of their social world. Individual men are not puppets of an abstract 'society' or even of a 'patriarchy', but benefit from women's oppression personally and specifically. They may or may not promote patriarchal ideas equally personally. I don't think the kind of theory which attempts to gloss over this can get any grip on the day-to-day realities of relations between the sexes.

In this chapter I look only at this culture. As we have seen, most theories, including many feminist theories about menstruation, emphasise the idea that 'menstrual taboos are universal' (e.g. Weideger, 1978), and then go on to talk about 'other cultures', treating them as somehow a more extreme version of 'us'. I think that each culture should be examined in its specificity – if this were to be done, I would expect the fact to emerge that menstruation is actually used very flexibly to express a considerable range of ideas about woman's nature or place.

I look at this culture because it is my own, which I think gives me a better chance of understanding it, and also because I think there is something racist about the way in which 'our' men are never made the focus of attention. Constant references to Islam or to Orthodox Judaism and their supposedly excessive ways, presents our culture as normal – moderate, and even rational about 'these things'.

Women and men produce ideas about menstruation, and these ideas often come into conflict. I have looked first at men's ideas because I believe that men have social power over women, and therefore male definitions will tend to predominate within the culture. For the same reasons, the male perspective is more accessible to the researcher than a 'female' one.

The various data I will quote from here were gathered for my thesis on the social meanings of menstruation. In order to generate ideas about men's view of menstruation, I interviewed 14 white, relatively well-educated men, whose ages ranged from 21 to 40, and also taped a discussion in a 'men's group'. It is not easy to define a men's group (cf Bradshaw, 1982). They have grown up since the early 1970s among men who have been affected or influenced by feminist ideas. Some have called themselves 'men's liberation' groups, others 'men against sexism' groups – this particular one had not taken up either of these definitions. The interview sample was gathered in snowball fashion, through friendship networks, mostly from among men known to have an interest in sexual politics. My sample is not representative of any population: rather I hope it can give us some idea of how some men who are relatively familiar with feminist ideas understand menstruation.

I will first present a summary of the range of processes I think are involved in these men's view of menstruation, and then I will look in more depth at two aspects of this: firstly male culture, and secondly the etiquette of menstruation. By male culture I mean, essentially, what men say to other men, usually in exclusively male groups. This term inevitably slips somewhat into a larger notion of the sexist culture of a patriarchal society which includes women, for it is a feature of patriarchal societies that men-only groups hold positions of power within them. Ideas which are formed in male groups will therefore be present in 'mixed' contexts, although they may then be opposed by women. I am concentrating on the culture of male groups because I think women often underestimate its influence.

How men define menstruation

Menstruation is an aspect of women's bodies which is of no benefit to men, indeed which is 'naturally' unrelated to men. It is understood as one aspect of the sex difference. Men maintain their social power over women in part through an ideology which defines women as inferior to men, and as naturally fitting into the place men have designed for them. This includes universal heterosexuality and in many cultures, universal motherhood. The sex hierarchy is also expressed and reinforced by an elaborate etiquette which regulates relations between the sexes. In our culture, menstruation is not especially emphasised, but male definitions nevertheless prevent women from generating positive self/woman-centred understandings of it for themselves.

Patriarchal ideology is produced and sustained in a variety of ways. Male groups produce a sexist culture which contains reference to menstruation – jokes which men see as 'sick', which centre upon sex during menstruation, often linking it with violence. They accuse women of 'using' periods to 'get out of things' – defining this as an illegitimate use of power on women's part.

Medical men, especially gynaecologists, produce another important kind of ideology about women. They emphasise women's reproductive role as the only hope of health for women. Menstrual disorders are seen as the result of refusal to conform to the female role. Medicine institutionalises men's failure to empathise with female suffering and justifies it with the notion that inconvenient women's problems are 'psychosomatic' – that is, imaginary (cf Lennane and Lennane, 1973). Doctors frequently ascribe a woman's problems to her mother's influence, suggesting that mothers inculcate 'unhealthy' attitudes into their daughters. They seek to persuade women to place their trust in male authority, not in female support. Some female experiences can be distorted to fit men's ideas about women's inferiority – for example women's experiences of physical and mental changes during the menstrual cycle have been named 'premenstrual tension', and used to put women down as unreliable and out of control of their behaviour (Laws, 1983b and forthcoming).

Individual men are able then to use the various elements within the ideology to manipulate individual relationships with women to their own advantage. Present day British culture on menstruation and sexuality gives men the choice as to whether or not to engage in sexual intercourse during menstruation – women are not so free to make this choice since to initiate sex with a man is to risk a reaction of disgust, and to refuse sex can produce resentment and labelling as 'uptight'.

The etiquette of menstruation decrees that women may not make men aware of the existence of menstruation, either in general or in the particular. There is however no sanction against men referring to it. For example, women very rarely mention menstruation in the workplace even to excuse themselves because of menstrual pain. But men often explain women's behaviour when they disapprove of it as the result of 'the time of the month'.

Women do not as a matter of course refer to their own periods in public, feeling a sense of embarrassment or even shame at the thought of doing so. These feelings have often been discussed as though they were spontaneous, springing from something in the woman's own mind – I will try to show here how women's silences about their bodies result from fear of ridicule and harrassment by men. We will see that this fear is perfectly rational when we look at the experience of a group of women who disobeyed the etiquette. Women in this country who have attempted to publicly challenge the discriminatory taxation of sanitary wear have been alternately mocked and ignored, effectively kept out of the public sphere (Laws, 1983a). Men find reference to sanitary wear highly offensive. In a culture which tolerates a high street trade in moving pictures of the sexual torture of women, grown men reported to me feeling shock at seeing packets of tampons in women's bathrooms. The consequence of this etiquette is that in dealing with their periods, women are obliged to be constantly aware of men.

Knowledge of a woman's menstruation becomes something specially reserved for the heterosexual relationship: it must be kept carefully hidden from all other men including one's father and one's sons. Thus the experience of menstruation is reconstructed in such a way as to emphasise an image of women's lives as circumscribed by men's gaze – even while men themselves may be very little concerned with the matter.

In setting out the sexist ways in which menstruation is defined by men, I want to make it clear that I do not imagine there to be some simple alternative, a spontaneous, 'positive', female view of menstruation. Women's experiences of periods vary greatly, and are, of course, socially moulded. But it must be possible for women to refuse to allow men to use our physical characteristics against us without needing to romanticise them as somehow inherently glorious.

This chapter concentrates on male culture and I am presenting here only part of my data – often the men I interviewed are themselves reporting other men's behaviour. Where individual men had knowledge of male culture, this formed only a (larger or smaller) part of their consciousness of menstruation. The general picture was more one of competing influences, of confused and inconsistent sets of ideas. These ideas came from many sources – from other men but also from women (mothers, wives, friends), from women's magazines, from medical sources, from feminist writings – and the men had variously made more or less sense of what they had heard.

What men say to men

Why is it necessary, then, for us to concern ourselves with what men say to each other about women? If we are to understand the relations between the sexes, we must look at all social settings, not only the ones in which women are normally welcome. There exists in our society a whole range of men-only groupings which exclude women and within which male supremacist ideology goes unchallenged – this must have an influence on the way men see women in the rest of their lives.

Mary Daly calls this talk 'spooking from the locker room'. She writes that:

> . . . most of the time this language is used in all-male environments. Yet it is the common male view of all women and, although most women do not hear it directly, we receive the message in a muted way. It is conveyed through silences, sneers, jeers, excessive politeness, paternalistic praise and disapproval, aggressive physical contact (an arm around the shoulder, a pat on the behind), invasive stares. Since women often do not *hear* the messages of obscenity directly, we are spooked. For the invasive presence and the intent are both audible and inaudible, visible and invisible. (1978, p. 323) (Emphasis in original)

The reason I began researching menstruation was because I did not find that my own experience of it made sense to me – I felt there was information I did not have about it. I had not known that the kind of talk I describe here existed and, although in many ways I regret the knowledge, it does explain something of the atmosphere I had picked up around the subject.

About half of the men I interviewed recalled some sort of talk among men about menstruation – about the same numbers recalled such talk from childhood as from adult life. Among boys, the most common form of joking is about sanitary towels, calling them 'jam rags', or variants of this: 'jam roll', 'jam sandwich', etc.

> For years and years, I'm not the only person I'm sure, we used to . . . kids used to call, used to taunt girls, we used to say 'well, where's your jammy rags?' and things like that . . . people never knew what it was until I was older, but it's one of the things you just say . . . a way of getting at girls to do that. (interview 6)

Only a few men mentioned taunting girls like this – more often they said that such talk was among boys:

> A lot of men, a lot of the boys, used to have jokes, a pattern, a section of jokes about menstruation, like 'sunny periods' and all sorts of connotations about, um, there was a whole sort of part of the vocabulary of, like, jokes which were menstrual jokes
> SL: Would they say that to the girls?
> – No, that would be boys' jokes . . . But I can't really remember men's jokes being geared to persecuting one girl in particular, it was more sort of 'it's us and them, and they have periods, so we've got a few jokes about that sort of thing'. Bit like Irish, Pakistanis . . . (interview 10)

Several men said that such references would have been avoided as 'in bad taste' at their schools.

Girls also use slang and make jokes about periods – but I would argue that even the same words have a rather different meaning in female mouths. I certainly wouldn't think that taking a solemn attitude to periods would do girls any good!

Laughing at one's own bodily functions and the inconveniences they bring with them is a healthy sign and quite different from the 'them and us' joking of boys. That the man quoted above did not even know what was referred to by 'jammy rags', but knew that it was something he could say to 'get at girls', demonstrates my point. He understood the sexual politics without understanding the subject matter.

Adult joking usually seems to have other themes, although there is considerable overlap. The most common kind of joking among adult men seems to centre on sexual access, and this is also found in school-age males:

> . . . looking back at school, that's the kind of jokes you would make, if you ever sort of managed to get off with some girl it would be just your luck if she'd be having her period or whatever. (interview 11)

One man explained to me that he did not think he was representative of men generally because:

> I think a lot of men will use it as a derogatory term . . . from previous experience, they'll say 'Well she was fucking have her period, wasn't she?' Meaning they didn't have sex. 'She wasn't feeling very well', as though she did it on purpose to spite him or something. A lot of men think in those terms . . . (interview 8)

> When I was younger, you know, you used to say 'oh, hard luck' kind of thing, (laughs) 'picked the wrong one' that kind of thing (laughs). (interview 6)

In this discourse, women exist only for men's sexual use. Women are described as a class, defined as interchangeable in their sexual relation to men: a man may 'pick the wrong one'.

One man spelt out what he thought were the implications of this sort of talk when I asked him about whether menstruation featured in the pornography which he had told me was passed around on the engineering shop floor where he had worked:

> No, that's totally unerotic in male conceptions. Yeah, I mean the idea that . . . you know? It's just a turn off, for men. The jokes that men make about it are sort of like sick jokes you'd make, about Thalidomide dogs being taken for a drag, or something, the same sort of inference that it's a sick joke, you know, menstruation is a sick business, you know.
> SL: It isn't exactly that the women are sick, is it?
> – No, it's more like women, in a group of human beings, are redundant, when they're thought about in association with menstruation. That women and menstruation aren't erotic, you know, you don't sort of talk about them to stimulate a conversation, like. (interview 10)

This apparent absolute acceptance of the idea that sex does not take place during menstruation seems to co-exist with a kind of bravado, where stories are told about other men who do have sex with menstruating women.

> . . . there was this thing about grabbing hold of the tampon string with your teeth and dragging it out. It was really sort of getting high on . . . on the perverted . . . well trying to make sex during menstruation looked perverted and therefore get high on it. (interview 7)

This man told a story about his boss, when he worked in a hospital laboratory:

> . . . there was a female toilet just outside the lab so we could always see the women going to the toilet and he actually used to time them and if they were taking a long time he used to say 'oh well they've got the rags up, there's no point in chatting her up'. (interview 7)

Another theme of male talk about menstruation is that women 'use' it to get out of things. I first came across this in a university interview where a man suggested to me that this would be an important question for me to look at – 'how women use it'. One man talks about this in response to a question about menstrual pain:

> . . . I can remember that that was often a male reaction to period pains, that it was something that was completely not understandable, that it was something that was, that shouldn't happen, so therefore, men tended to think that it didn't happen, that it was something that women made up, to get out of things. I can remember feeling irritated, feeling annoyed, feeling that there was nothing . . . that I didn't have any control over the situation, and that it was something that women used to exert control. (interview 14)

Finally, we have the idea that something to do with the menstrual cycle makes women moody, bad-tempered, unreliable – men told me of this being said both about the time of the actual bleeding, and of 'PMT'. Often this was referred to as 'the time of the month', which makes it unnecessary to be exact about *which* time of the month is meant.

> SL: Would the women (at work) ever have said if they had periods, or anything about it?
> – No, but it usually became evident . . . . Because of, er well, whether it was actually evident or whether it was an imagined, imagined that it was, like they were in a bad mood and I think you imagined it because it was their period . . . Because mainly in my job, it tended to be the women that did it, I was always in a minority, either on my own or with one or two others. And so if there were a lot of women there'd obviously be someone who was in a bad mood because they were menstruating, at least that's what we put it down to.
> SL: Is that all of you or you men, put it down to, do you think? I mean, what would the women say to each other?
> – No, I mean it was not discussed with the women. Um, maybe sometimes we'd overhear women saying 'oh, she's in a bad mood, but it's that time of the month', so they'd sort of forgive her, or . . . But I think it was mainly to do with the men. And even, maybe because I'd worked with other men and we'd talking around

> that, that you know, 'oh she's in a bad mood she's bloody menstruating again' (laughs) you know, er, when I worked on my own with women I still had that mentality, that you know, 'jesus christ, who's menstruating again?' (laughs) (interview 7)

I see this kind of joking talk among men as a process of policing the periphery.

As far as I can learn, menstruation is never referred to in pornography, which could be called a representation of the male-centred ideal of sexuality. In the most purely male fantasies of woman, then, periods simply do not exist.

The impression given from the men I talked to, was that this joking goes on most intensely in men-only situations which are close to mixed situations, where men pass between the two. The shop floor where men go home to their wives is one case, the weekend football team's dressing room is another. Men who had been to boys-only schools were much less likely to remember joking about periods. It is as if such verbal attacks on women as a group are needed as part of the process of re-establishing the particular power of the male group. When men need to interact with women as individuals every day, the male group must redefine itself against women as a mass.

In the course of doing this work I was repeatedly made aware that I was asking to be told things women are not meant to hear. Some of the men themselves became aware of this. One said at one point, 'Sorry I'm being so upfront about it. Do you find that offensive?' (interview 10), and another almost apologised for what he was telling me: 'I have to be frank' (interview 7). These two were the men who gave me the fullest accounts of male culture. Several of the other men said they could not remember the content of jokes or words, although they said they remembered them being told. One responded to my prompting him for details like this: 'Yes. Not sure if we can talk further about that. I don't know what sort of area you're interested in . . . ' (interview 2).

My impression was very much that these were sexual insults which are meant to be kept among men, and that for men to tell them to me created unease in the interviews. It was interesting that, although several of the men told me quite personal details of their sexual experiences, and of relationships, nothing created the same sort of awkwardness as my asking to hear 'men's talk'. A number of the men responded to my questioning with references to 'the sort of things boys say', 'in the schoolboy sense' or would just say 'you know', appealing to a common sense knowledge I did not have. What made the men anxious was not my hearing about their personal feelings, but about their participation in male groups which talk about women in this way.

This brings us, conveniently, to etiquette: what may and may not be said and done, in what settings, by whom, and to whom.

The etiquette of menstruation

Looking at male culture, my feeling was of discovery – that I was learning about things I had not known. In contrast, trying to describe the etiquette around menstruation is a matter of making systematic knowledge one already has, but in an inexplicit way.

Etiquette is defined by Edward Norbeck (following Leslie White) as 'rules of behaviour governing social relations among people of distinct social statuses or classes, hierarchical and non-hierarchical' (Norbeck, 1977, p. 72). In this article 'A Sanction for Authority: Etiquette', he argues that taboo should be seen as a special class of the larger category of etiquette, 'as rules of etiquette to which supernatural sanctions are attached' (p. 73). He then concentrates on pre-modern Japanese and Polynesian rules of behaviour, to show how intensely hierarchical social structures are served by such rules. However, he also suggests that etiquette is important in modern societies, perhaps especially in relation to defining and preserving the social statuses of women and men, where it continues to 'reflect and support formal and informal relations of authority' (p. 73).

This gives us an interesting perspective on the way in which the term 'taboo' is used in much of the modern discourse on menstruation. It is frequently used to refer to *any* kind of social recognition of menstruation – this leaves one vaguely searching for the missing supernatural sanction. 'Taboo' is simply the wrong word for what takes place in our culture.

Let us try to lay out the basic shape of our culture's menstrual etiquette – since these rules are generally not made explicit, this is very much a matter of reading absences. The rule behind all the others seems to be that women may not draw men's attention to menstruation in any way. This is most intensely enforced in the public world, for in private men may agree to waive the rules within a particular relationship. Some kind of distinction between public and private was a theme which came up repeatedly in my data. For instance one man says in the group discussion:

> When you first come across someone who is menstruating who you're close to . . . Even though I knew all the mechanics of it, and I understood the thing, it seemed, you know, like a source of worry, because all the taboos had been about women in general, they hadn't been about a particular woman . . . (men's group)

To look first at public settings, I asked the men I interviewed whether they had heard reference to menstruation at work. Among all of them, with many years of working life between them, they could remember only three or four instances of women saying that they were off work because of menstrual pain. Where this had happened, it was in somewhat unusual workplaces: from students in a university, and from women in a particularly relaxed and friendly social work office.

They reported no instance of a woman referring to mood changes related to menstruation in a public setting. And yet several of them said that remarks about the 'time of the month', as we have seen, are commonplace among men in some workplaces. This is, of course, related to ideas about menopause – it would be very discrediting in most situations for a woman to refer to her own menopausal symptoms, and yet men will speak of older women as affected by the 'time of life'.

An exception to the rule brings out an interesting response in the man concerned. One man described an instance of reference to sanitary wear in a public setting – a canteen where he had worked as a very young man.

> There were about thirty women, . . . and they did talk about lots of things, in front of each other, which I didn't, I didn't have any . . . I used to get taunted as well, lots of sexual innuendo . . . The women used to talk about their periods, they're coming on next week, or . . . and . . .
> SL: Did you find that embarrassing?
> – Um . . . yes, because there were so many women together, talking about it and, it was an experience I didn't have, and didn't particularly understand either, really, and I'd usually walk out of the room or walk away from them, try not to listen.
> SL: Would they be ignoring you, then, or trying to get at you?
> – They weren't particularly ignoring me, they were just talking about it. (interview 6)

Here the women are in the great majority, and the man is low status. Note that he does what he can to change the situation, he finds it disturbing that the women are disregarding the etiquette, even though he recognises that there is no aggressive intent there.

Other transgressions are more deliberate. Some of the women antinuclear protesters at Greenham Common have tied tampons to the wire of the perimeter fence. A friend told me that her father had been so shocked by this that he could hardly speak about it. I found another interesting example in a recent review of Gloria Steinem's new book, *Outrageous Acts and Everyday Rebellions*:

> Despite her book's title, Gloria Steinem's talent is not for outrage. That she should leave to Germaine Greer, who she remembers taunting a talk-show host by demanding, as he laid down the law about monthly emotional changes and female unreliability, 'Can you tell me if I'm menstruating right now – or not?' (Conrad, 1984)

No-one is telling any stories about the outrageousness of the talk-show host, who raised the topic.

What then, of private life? Only a few of the men I interviewed had ever heard their mothers talk about menstruation – most had seen no evidence of it. More than one of them was quite startled by the thought that their mothers must have menstruated. Half of those who had sisters had heard no mention of their periods – this includes one man who had six sisters. In adult sexual relationships, on the other hand, the men would on the whole know when the women were menstruating. Indeed this knowledge in a sense marks off the heterosexual relationship from all other relationships between the sexes. However, one man told about a girlfriend he had been involved with some time ago:

> . . . I used to see sanitary towels lying around, and I used to tell her to put them away . . .
> SL: Oh did you . . . you thought they shouldn't be . . . ?
> – Well, yeah, I don't know I just didn't want them to be hanging around, lying around . . . (interview 6)

Other men tell about seeing packets of sanitary wear which were not hidden as important moments in changing their consciousness about menstruation:

> It was quite a shock for me in later years to walk into toilets and see packets of Tampax and things . . . before I had any conception, like, of the women's movement . . . It was a real shock, you know, even though I . . . the initial feelings were shock, and then I thought, no point in being shocked . . . (interview 10)

> . . . One of the big surprises of adult life, was going into people's houses and finding things openly displayed in places. I couldn't believe it, because at home these things had always been hidden away, and it was like a real shock to me, because it was like something that was not mentioned, never spoken about . . . (men's group)

Notice that women generally offend against this code of omission. Men's sense of what is due to them as men is upset by women not observing the etiquette of concealment fully.

Etiquette within the heterosexual relationship

The etiquette of sexual relationships has the same structure as the general one – that is, it expresses and maintains the social statuses of women and of men. Basically women must behave as if menstruation was offensive to the man, until he convincingly gives her permission to assume otherwise. One man describes this situation from his perspective:

Yeah . . . yes I feel that quite a few women, if I were, if a man were to say to them that he, that they were in favour of having sex when they thought that their partner was also in favour of having sex when they were menstruating, that the women would feel that they were saying that in spite of their real feelings . . .
SL: Yes, I can see that . . . they'd be so sure that it really was . . .
– Repulsive . . . Yes I'm sure there's one end of the spectrum of attitudes by men which that does hold true for, but I don't think it's as pervasive as a lot of women think. (interview 9)

Men also report that women are typically more anxious than they are about staining the sheets and so on:

She's actually more preoccupied than I am . . . I mean at a practical level, I think it's *reasonable* to stop things getting stained, I do actually, I appreciate in some ways, her taking care of that, being careful in that sense. But I suspect it's also careful partly in the sense of kind of protecting herself and slightly hiding herself away. And I respect that, and I don't want to push her, in that way, so it may be that in one sense I feel less exposed to the existence of the blood and its flow than I might be. (interview 12)

. . . quite often far more embarrassment in the women, well certainly in me, because I've sort of lost that taboo quite some time ago . . .
– Certainly some women that I've slept with have been totally embarrassed by having a period, and that's actually because of prior experience, and I've said, look it doesn't bother me, if it bothers you, then, fair enough . . .
– most people check it out, don't they? (men's group)

Obviously this has something to do with who does the washing, but I think there is also a sense that even if the rule against sex during periods is disregarded, women still have to somehow protect men from their female bodies. This expectation also comes out in a discussion of the smell of menstrual blood, which took place in the men's group.

It emerges that a number of the men in the group feel quite happy about what they call 'making love', that is 'normal' sex, during periods, but most of them are anxious about what they call 'oral sex' (male to female, that is). They discuss whether or not they would in fact be able to taste or smell the blood, and some try to reassure others that 'it doesn't involve that much blood'. I did not ask the men I interviewed about this, but in the men's group, where I did not set the agenda, the men returned several times to the question of the smell of menstrual blood.

Shere Hite's survey of men's attitudes towards sex also uncovered considerable preoccupation with the idea that women's genitals smell bad. A number of men felt that women should wash before sex:

> – Cunnilingus stinks! The smell is horrendous!
> – How does one ask a woman politely to wash?
> – If I want to have oral sex with a gal, I am saying to her, 'You are clean' (Hite, 1981, pp. 688–9)

As Hite points out, no man mentioned the need to brush teeth before kissing. I would say this could be seen as a demand for women to observe an etiquette of purity on approaching men's bodies. Would the men reciprocate, I wonder? What is conveyed is that women can't assume that their bodies are acceptable just as they are.

What I found in relation to sex was that some of the men I talked with were interested in changing the categories of what is and is not allowed by the etiquette of menstruation, to allow what they define as 'sex' during that time.

When they talked about sex during periods, what seemed to interest them was breaking rules, not ignoring them or doing away with them:

> I think I thought it was . . . no, not dirty, . . . I think I thought that it was exciting, you know, that we were sort of breaking some rule . . . that particular rule was broken along with a whole lot of other rules at the same time, . . . it developed in terms of what I was thinking about things in general. (interview 14)

In the group, one man says how he finds sex more exciting during menstruation than at other times:

> Does my experience . . . ?
> – Yes, it rings bells, yes . . .
> – It does for me . . . but like we talked about before, for me at least part of it, is to do with the unacceptability of periods, right from being little . . . I mean that was all sorts of things. Like touching or looking at, well anybody's genitals, it wasn't on . . . and that makes the idea of doing so quite interesting. And periods were really sort of beyond the pale, you know that's almost a last barrier in not-allowed behaviour, which is now OK, and I think that adds an extra . . . it's a forbidden fruit thing, I think.
> – I suppose that was what was obscenely attractive about that Hells Angels thing.[1]
> – mm, right
> – . . . that you're actually, they'd really done what was the most taboo of things, and there's perhaps unfortunately something slightly erotic about that. (men's group)

The impulse here seems to be directed against an older generation which is perceived as repressive – but it does not transcend the old rules, it depends upon them.

It also became clear that this 'issue' of sex during periods was *the* issue about menstruation for many of the men – which places the whole experience into a sexual context which is not the context that women tend to see it in. The sexualisation of menstruation becomes a problem in itself.

Although, as we see, they view their own behaviour as coming out of social conventions, the men I talked to perpetually referred to the behaviour of women they were involved with in individualised terms. One man said about a woman he had recently become involved with who was embarrassed by an incident which made it plain to him that she was menstruating that 'it's obviously a block that she's got, because in every other respect she is not the least bit embarrassed'. For himself, 'again *I* didn't feel any sort of problem with that, at all'. (interview 1) Women's concern for etiquette is understood as evidence of some sort of personal hang-up.

Etiquette, male culture and men's power over women

Beginning to draw the threads of this chapter together, let us look at what the etiquette of menstruation implies about what talk between the sexes may occur. As we have seen, men on occasion refer to periods in a derogatory way in front of women. But do men discuss it with women friends?

> . . . for instance in conversation, I've got lots of friends who are quite open about sexual matters, sexual politics, but still I don't, wouldn't talk to women about it. I certainly wouldn't initiate a conversation about it, I'm sure. (laughs quietly) (interview 6)

> . . . depending on the circumstances . . . would need a bit of warming up to discuss that topic, it wasn't the kind of, walk in, 'How's your period?' kind of discussion (laughs). No, I mean it just seems ludicrous to . . . And presumably would be quite rightly resented . . . But also the other side is, I wouldn't initiate a discussion . . . (interview 2)

This understanding that for a man to raise the topic would not be in the woman's interests must I think refer back to their own sex's version of menstruation – as entirely discrediting. The construction of menstruation as 'women's affair' interlocks with the perception that reference to menstruation from men to women is generally threatening. Part of what encourages women to comply with the elaborate and inconvenient etiquette I have tried to describe, is the fear of provoking such reference, such humiliation.

An interesting case of an instance where women have deliberately acted against the etiquette of menstruation and have tried to bring an issue related to menstruation to public attention, is the campaign against Value Added Tax on sanitary wear which has existed in this country for the last few years. I interviewed the women who have been most involved about the reactions they had met with in their work (Laws, 1983a).

The issue has been raised in Parliament on a few occasions, and male MPs have invariably treated it as a joke. The campaigners have also had a lot of trouble getting journalists to report on it: Denise Flowers, the campaign's co-ordinator, describes the attitude as one of 'hilarity and dismissal'. Often an initial contact has been positive, but after the journalist has gone back to his or her office and mentioned it, they never hear anything again. At one point a journalist on the *Times* wanted to publish a letter on the subject, but his editor refused, saying he was not having the words 'sanitary towel' in the *Times*.

On a few occasions they have been met with outright sexual harrassment – Denise Flowers was bothered by an obscene telephone caller for 18 months after her name was mentioned in a local paper. When she called in to one 'phone-in programme on Capital Radio, the men who answered the 'phone made her listen to a looped tape which detailed the symptoms of venereal diseases – as they said, this was to show her how 'poxy' they thought her cause was. On both these occasions the authorities were totally unhelpful when Denise complained.

The reactions of men in public life to this campaign were consistent with the themes of male culture as it relates to menstruation which I learnt about from my interviews and the group discussion. Exactly as Leslie White describes in his general discussion of etiquette, it is enforced by 'social sanctions, such as adverse comment or criticism, ridicule, and ostracism' (White, 1959, p. 225).

From a conservative position, White spells out nicely for me the importance of etiquette:

> . . . many persons who do not understand the nature and functions of systems of etiquette are inclined to rail against them as being irrational, senseless and therefore unnecessary. They fail to understand that society must have some way of assuring itself that men will behave as men, women as women. (White, 1959, p. 226)

Using the example of a male student who arrives in class wearing lipstick or earrings, he emphasises 'the significant and important point: we do not know what he will do next' (White, 1959). It is interesting that White uses examples from sexual politics to illustrate his point, though he does not remark on this. Etiquette is clearly a particularly characteristic feature of the social hierarchy of the sexes – we take it for granted so much that it is difficult to see it for what it is.

I hope that this chapter will be useful to feminist analysis beyond the specific subject of menstruation. In interviewing men I have tried to change the focus of my investigation to avoid the danger of victim-blaming which can arise in work done 'on women'. I have suggested that the culture of men-only groups may be an essential subject to study in attempting to understand women's situation, even where the influence of such groups is indirect, and have described some of the problems of such research for women.

In seeking terms to describe the treatment of menstruation in our culture, I have rejected the use of 'taboo' as inappropriate and confusing. Women researching incest have also challenged the common use of the notion of taboo, pointing out that father–daughter incest is in fact neither very uncommon, nor effectively sanctioned in patriarchal society (Rush, 1981). I have suggested that 'etiquette' is a more suitable word for the way that menstruation is handled in this culture, but we should also be alerted to the way in which the notion of taboo may obscure social power relations which women need to see clearly.

To sum up what I have been saying about menstruation: I would see the culture of male groups as one important institution enforcing and generating male-supremacist definitions of menstruation. Etiquette is one procedure by which women's compliance with these definitions is policed. Hiding the existence of periods forces women to be endlessly aware of men's potential presence, their gaze entering even the most private and mundane parts of a woman's life. And, if women may not speak in public about periods, they are blocked from generating new understandings of their bodies which could challenge men's.

Women enact their acceptance of men's definitions by complying with the etiquette. And rebel by breaking it. I have mentioned some examples of explicit rebellion against the etiquette of menstruation. Others can be seen where feminists implicitly make the connection between refusing such etiquette and refusing male domination, and call a magazine *Red Rag*, a cartoon book *Heavy Periods*, a theatre piece *Female Trouble* and a rock band *PMT*.

There is no need, then, to resort to the unconscious or to any abstract notion of 'society' to explain social attitudes towards menstruation. They can be accounted for as part of the process by which men maintain their social power over women.

Note

1. Several men in the group had heard in their schooldays about Hells Angels having sex with menstruating women as one of their rituals of defilement.

3 The Hidden Pathology of the Male Reproductive System

Naomi Pfeffer

Women as patients are more visible than men since they visit doctors frequently for all conditions and especially those associated with reproduction, so much so that it has been argued that 'women do more than "enter" the health care system through their reproductive organs, they often organise their health care around gynaecological care' (Ruzek, 1979, p. 11). Men consult doctors less frequently and present them with a different range of conditions so that, as Marieskind suggests, 'we would think it very humorous to have men entering the health system through their penises, reproductive systems and urologists' (Marieskind, 1975, p. 48).

Several explanations have been offered for the different health experiences of men and women. One explanation which is well-rehearsed locates the difference in biology; it claims that women's greater consultation rates for conditions relating to reproduction arise because women's reproductive systems are structurally vulnerable, their functions exacting a great physical price. Men, in contrast, have reproductive systems which operate with mechanical ease and efficiency with few detrimental effects.

Simone de Beauvoir in the first chapter of *The Second Sex*, exemplifies this approach. She locates the difference between the sexes in their reproductive functions. From foetus to old age 'the development of the male is comparatively simple' (de Beauvoir, 1972, p. 58) whereas for the female 'this whole occurrence has the aspect of a crisis' (de Beauvoir, 1972, p. 59) and 'instability is strikingly characteristic of women's organisation in general' (de Beauvoir, 1972, p. 60). De Beauvoir believes that a woman suffers from 'infirmity in the abdomen' (de Beauvoir, 1972, p. 63) because she is 'the theatre of a play that unfolds within her in which she is not personally concerned' (de Beauvoir, 1972, p. 60). This play has nothing to do with her personal survival, but is acted out for the benefit of the egg and hence the species. This 'conflict between species and individual, which sometimes assumes dramatic force at childbirth, endows the feminine body with a disturbing frailty' (de Beauvoir, 1972, p. 63). Spermatogenesis and coition, however, 'rob the male of little vitality' (de Beauvoir, 1972, p. 64) and 'in comparison with her, the male seems infinitely favoured: his sexual life is not in opposition to his existence as a person, and biologically, it runs an even course, without crises and generally without mishap' (de Beauvoir, 1972, p. 64).

Some feminists have challenged explanations which imply that theories of male superiority must ultimately rest on biology. Instead they claim that the definition of women as biologically vulnerable and unhealthy is a social construction formulated in male terms, instrumental in the subordination of women by men (Sayers, 1982, p. 3; Ehrenreich and English, 1973, p. 9). They point to the ways in which normal reproductive functions have become 'medicalised', that is, defined as medical problems (Oakley, 1976b; Rich, 1977a; Leeson and Gray, 1978). To counteract this, they recommend a redefinition of women's reproductive health in which 'normal' processes are no longer seen as pathological. Any difficulties experienced by women are due, they claim, to the ways in which men have organised the world to suit themselves, often at the expense of women (Sayers, 1982, p. 25). Women are encouraged to adopt a celebratory attitude towards their bodies and to rejoice in their unique reproductive functions, menstruation, childbirth and the menopause (Daly, 1978, p. 60). Running alongside this challenge is a feminist critique of medicine which argues that medicine overlooks or discounts as trivial women's genuine complaints about conditions associated with reproduction such as premenstrual tension, dysmenorrhea, vaginal infections and cystitis (Elston, 1981, p. 194).

Negotiating this contradiction can lead to confusion. What is or is not a legitimate female reproductive disorder? What medicine describes as abnormal, feminists claim is 'normal', and vice versa. Sedgwick points out that 'disease models are equally the inventive constructions of the mind which may be more or less firmly based in empirical evidence and theoretical elegance' (Sedgwick, 1982, p. 31). This observation applies equally to medical and feminist definitions of female reproductive pathology. The contradiction arises, I believe, because the efforts of feminists to unmask the role of medicine as an instrument of social control have focused solely on definitions and treatment of women. Not only does this strategy lead to confusion about the nature of reproductive pathology, but it also leads to feminists fighting half the battle. For if medicine is instrumental in the subordination of women by defining them as weak, so too is it instrumental in the superordination of men by defining them as strong. Implicit in the medical definitions and unchallenged by feminists, is the assumption that the male reproductive system is structurally efficient, and that its functions proceed smoothly. In this chapter I will challenge that assumption. I will argue that whilst medicine highlights the potential for reproductive disorders in women, it makes them invisible in men. As Ruth Hubbard suggests 'we need to construct a more inclusive and, in that sense, truer reality by pulling forth facts that have previously been ignored, while pushing back others which have received more notoriety than their substance merits' (Hubbard, 1981, p. 217).

Following the format of structure and function, I will discuss first the assumptions made about the reproductive systems of men and women, and then I will outline the ways in which the efficiency of both systems is described by examining measures of fertility. I have drawn on medical sources and those of reproductive physiology which inform much of medical knowledge.

Structure: reproductive systems

Dale Spender claims that language has the power to shape reality so that once categories are constructed within language, we proceed to organise the world according to those categories (Spender, 1980, p. 2). In *Man Made Language*, Dale Spender cites linguistic research which found more positive words for males and many negative words for females which have no equivalent for males (Spender, 1980, p. 15). Thus, through language, the image of one sex, the male, is enhanced, whilst that of the female is diminished. The language of reproductive medicine is no exception to this finding.

What does the language of fertility tell us about ourselves? The bias in the information given by medical textbooks on reproduction has been well illustrated in articles such as 'A funny thing happened on the way to the Orifice' (Scully and Bart, 1978), in which Diana Scully and Pauline Bart analyse the ways in which women and their sexuality are represented to medical students through textbook information which confirms the view of women as incapable of sexual response, whose sole role and source of fulfilment is as wife and mother. Such analyses consider the content of the information presented but not the language used.

There is a whole host of negative words in medicine to describe the female reproductive system. A woman can suffer from *irregular* menstrual cycles caused by hormonal *imbalances* which can lead to *hostile* cervical mucus and *irregular* shedding of the lining of her uterus which may be structurally *retroverted*. If she does ovulate, she may fail to conceive because of *blocked* fallopian tubes. Or she may conceive an *ectopic* (*wrongly-placed*) pregnancy. Then she faces the danger of *spontaneous* or even *habitual* miscarriage due perhaps to a *blighted* ovum or even an *incompetent* cervix. And once she has given birth, her uterus may suffer *chronic subinvolution* and subsequently *prolapse*. The picture created is of a precarious, inefficient system.

For men, there are almost no negative terms; testicles may be undescended and the prostate may become inflamed or enlarged but the vocabulary which so negatively describes women is not available for men. Furthermore, any discussion of the male reproductive system moves rapidly away from the organs themselves and focuses on the quality of semen. Compare this with women where the health of the ovum is rarely discussed except to impute blame, and unreasonably so, in the case of miscarriage. And when the quality of semen is discussed, only positive terms are used. Human semen contains a high proportion of abnormally shaped, immotile sperm and their presence is used to assess the fertility of semen. This is expressed as the percentage normally shaped and motile, so that it is considered normal for an ejaculate to contain 60 per cent morphologically sound sperm and 60 per cent motile. The measures of fertility are expressed in positive terms and not as 40 per cent misshapen or 40 per cent immotile sperm.

Another strategy used shows that it is not necessary to state that the female system is more likely to have disorders than the male; by simply restricting interest to the disorders, fallibility is communicated. Consider the following chapter headings in a book titled *Systemic Pathology* (Payling Wright and Symmers, 1966):

Chapter 26. The Male Reproductive System.
Chapter 27. Gynaecological Pathology.

Both of these chapters discuss disease.

Positive terms for men and negative terms for women are found not only in the language of reproduction but in the concepts themselves. For instance, medicine tells us that the female reproductive system is more complicated than the male. 'The male reproductive tract has relatively simple functions being concerned almost exclusively with the production and transport of spermatozoa and it has none of the complex cyclical changes characteristic of the female' (Passmore and Robson, 1968, p. 24). I will take issue with this claim for three reasons.

Firstly, it is not based on equal levels of knowledge; far less is known about the male reproductive system than about the female. This is because 'research on the reproductive biology of the male has attracted far less attention than that of the female (and) serious gaps remain in our knowledge' (Fawcett, 1977, p. 355).

In descriptions of both the male and female reproductive systems, a factory metaphor is frequently used. In the male, the production process appears straightforward; the testicles are the plant producing sperm which are stored in the epididymis until they are needed whereupon they are transported by the vas deferens and urethra and delivered by the penis. But is this process as straightforward as descriptions would lead us to believe? Although the dependence of the male reproductive system on testosterone was demonstrated in 1946 by Moore and his colleagues (Fawcett, 1979, p. 556) and the presence of complex hormonal feedback systems is now recognised, how these affect reproductive function remains unexplained. Nor is the interaction between the sex organs understood. So reproductive structure and function in the male can be presented in simple terms. When something does go wrong, for example, when a man is found to be infertile, medicine extends the production metaphor to include the work environment; men are told that sperm damage is due to their testicles overheating either because of a variococele (a varicose vein in the testicles) impeding the natural cooling system, or tight underpants. Doctors prescribe a change of underwear and recommend that men spray their testicles with cold water (Speroff *et al.* 1979, p. 365).

In women, the production process appears much more complex because far more is known. The organs of reproduction are described as being functionally dependent and controlled by complex hormonal cycles. When reproductive function is impaired, a whole range of tests are available to locate the cause, either in the structure of the organs or in the controlling hormones (Speroff *et al.* 1979, pp. 314–33).

Secondly, where there is evidence of disease in the male reproductive organs, that disease is obscured. Unlike the female reproductive system, which is served by gynaecology, there is no medical specialty for the male reproductive system.

> Diseases of the female genital tract are numerous and extremely common in clinical and pathological practice, to the point at which they have been segregated into specialties unto themselves, in gynaecology and gynaecologic pathology. (Robbins, 1974, p. 1205)

Statements such as this make it easy to believe that the male reproductive system suffers almost no disease. Furthermore, when it does occur in men, it is possible for disease to remain unconnected to reproduction.

When a man has any problem with his reproductive organs, the medical specialist he consults is a urologist. That urologists should be concerned with the male reproductive system is seen as logical because the two systems, urination and reproduction, are intimately linked. Furthermore, the most common disorders of the male reproductive system present as problems of urination and not reproduction, for example, disorders of the prostate. The link with reproduction remains hidden. Consider a woman suffering backache because of a prolapse of her uterus; we would consider it odd if she were treated by an orthopaedic surgeon or osteopath and not a gynaecologist. In *Adam's Rib*, Ruth Herschberger points out that 'female trouble has been such a favourite joke with men that it would be painful to admit how often a man's trips to the urologist are prompted by aches and pains inhabiting the sex organs' (Herschberger, 1970, p. 66).

Prostatitis, inflammation of the prostate, the organ which produces the bulk of the seminal fluid, is called the 'silent disease' because it can be asymptomatic. 'Most men with chronic prostatitis have no reason to suspect it' (Smith, 1978, p. 170). Nevertheless, some enlargement of the prostate occurs in 30 to 50 per cent of men after age 50 and although conservative therapy is the recommended treatment, it is estimated that 1 in 10 men will require surgery (Smith, 1978, p. 289). The elderly prostate is frequently affected by benign or malignant neoplasm, and malignancy in the prostate is almost as common as malignancy of the lung and gastrointestinal tract. Whilst cancer of the prostate is the eighth largest cause of death in men (OPCS mortality statistics 1976) it is not always fatal. As Robbins tells us:

> There is a wide discrepancy between the frequency of carcinoma of the prostate as a clinical cause of disease and death and its prevalence as an anatomic lesion. (Robbins, 1974, p. 1196)

This prevalence is illustrated in a study where a series of autopsies were performed on men over age 80. It was found that two-thirds of these men had prostatic cancer (Smith, 1978, p. 290).

Amongst elderly men diseases of the prostate are so common that urologists urge routine screening, a simple procedure, so that silent chronic prostatitis and cancer of the prostate may be discovered and treated. If urologists believe that pathology of the prostate warrants more attention than it receives at present, we have to ask why these problems are not more widely recognised. On the other hand, diseases of the prostate rarely occur in men under age 50 (unlike cancer of the testis which is more common in younger, sexually active men). Diseases of the prostate are associated with declining hormone production and sexual inactivity. Perhaps this explains the lack of advertisement of its prevalence in men. It could be argued that disorders of the prostate are part of the 'normal' ageing process in men. As Armstrong points out in relation to ageing: 'age rendered the fundamental distinction between normal and pathological problematic' (Armstrong, n.d.). In women, disorders associated with the menopause and declining hormone production are treated with hormone replacement therapy. In this way, medicine treats the menopause as a 'deficiency disease'. Yet hormone replacement therapy, or any other therapy, is not offered to men, suggesting that unlike women, for men the processes of ageing are not deemed pathological.

How does treatment of the pathology of the reproductive organs differ in men and women? Because it is elderly men who have these diseases, the treatment offered is usually conservative, that is, no surgery, whereas the treatment offered women is more likely to be radical, that is, surgical removal of the diseased organs. Thus it would not be meaningful to compare the rate of, say, hysterectomy with prostatectomy, especially as it appears that many hysterectomies are performed as treatment for 'excessive menstruation' (Grant and Hussein, 1984). A comparison of surgical interventions would not therefore indicate that men experience as much, or less, disease of their reproductive organs as women.

Surgery or drug therapy for diseases of the male reproductive system can often lead to impotence and loss of sexual desire. In point, urologists appear to be no more sympathetic or understanding of sexual problems than gynaecologists, perhaps because those complaining are elderly men in whom sexual interest is considered inappropriate. For example, one urologist says:

> Impotence after transurethral resection of the prostate is clearly related to anxiety, old wives' tales and lack of explanation . . . post-operative impotence is associated with depressive states and in many cases the operation is clearly only one factor in a complicated psychosexual disorder. (Notley, 1979, p. 15)

Finally, as proof of its claim that the female reproductive system is more vulnerable than the male, medicine cites the greater number of functions performed by women's reproductive systems than men's. But it appears that a multiplicity of functions only leads to disease when these functions are specifically female. My textbook on biology tells me that the liver performs over 500 functions regulating the internal and chemical composition of the body which are essential to survival (Roberts, 1976, pp. 206–8). Yet the liver is not renowned for its tendency to break down. On the contrary, its ability to perform so many functions is marvelled at and it is described in glowing terms with copious use of adjectives such as 'remarkable', 'excellent', 'vital', etc. (Roberts, 1976). So while it is certainly true that the female reproductive system performs more functions than the male, that is menstruation, the nurturance and deliverance of a foetus, there is no clear reason why these should result in greater disease. And if a multiplicity of functions is highly valued in the liver, why is it not in the female reproductive system? It seems that despite her essential role in reproducing the species, the female is an exception to functional biology.

Function: the measures of fertility

There is a wide range of tests available to medicine to assess the fertility of a woman, reflecting both the greater knowledge of the female reproductive system and a willingness to intervene (Pfeffer and Woollett,

1983). Some tests examine the structure of the organs, others look at the hormonal controls. However, when a man has his status checked, the medical gaze rests cursorily on his organs of reproduction and only on those external to his body. Examination consists of assessing size, weight and position; physicians are advised to measure testicular size using an orchidometer, which comprises a number of metal balls of different sizes usually kept discretely in the doctor's pocket (Hudson and Burger, 1979). Why testicular size is used as an indicator is unclear, despite its apparent correlation with fertility in the bull! (Short, 1979). It reminds me of the nineteenth century anthropometric assumption that big equals better, so consequently brain size was taken as a measure of intellectual capacity (Mozans, 1974, p. 115).

Tests of male fertility are physically non-intrusive, unlike many of the procedures performed on women. Perhaps this reflects a universal tendency referred to by Margaret Walters in *The Male Nude*:

> though contemporary artists put the female body and genitals though the most fearful and drastic distortion, they tend to treat their own organs conservatively, gently, protectively. (Walters, 1979, p. 270)

However, the main test of male fertility focuses on measuring the quality of semen. Compare this to women where at no stage is the quality of the ovum checked. Once shed from the ovary, it is assumed that failure to conceive is due to some disorder elsewhere in her reproductive system. In practical terms semen is easier to collect than the ovum, but eggs can now be and are, retrieved from within the female pelvic cavity for in vitro fertilisation. This same procedure could be used to assess the fertility of the ovum if it was considered medically important. Furthermore, it is difficult to account for the difference in treatment of the gametes in purely pragmatic terms, because some of the tests of female fertility require the same surgical procedure as that used to retrieve eggs.

Fertility in men and women is unequivocally proven by the all-or-nothing fact of conception. In practice, the emphasis between the sexes differs:

> Fertility in mammals is determined by the absence or presence of a conceptus in a female. At any one time this all-or-nothing fact permits no gradations between these two extremes. Male fertility, on the other hand, depends in each instance *on the performance of the best-prepared gamete among millions of its fellows seminated.* (Salisbury *et al.* 1976, p. 222) (emphasis added)

Thus, female fertility is measured by an event, a conception, whereas fertility in males is conceptualised as fertilising capacity, a potential which is a property of sperm and which can be translated into a quantifiable, predictive measurement. These different measures of fertility assign a passive role to the female and an active role to the male in conception and thereby reproduce gender stereotypes. Thus the language and concepts available to describe reproductive processes, a process which lies at the heart of debates on gender differences, is itself gendered, making a feminist analysis of the steps involved well-nigh impossible. Ruth Herschberger tries to counteract what she describes as 'the painful persistent tendency to award the female a derogatory role' (Herschberger, 1970, p. 71). She offers a matriarchal account of biology and describes semen as laboriously put together by one doubtful function after another so that 'it begins to seem a miracle that it stays intact as long as it does' (Herschberger, 1970, p. 78). This matriarchal version of male biology however appears absurd because it violates our 'normal' patriarchally constructed conceptions, that is, of men being positive and women negative.

Unfortunately, there is no unanimity of what constitutes a fertile male. Consequently, we have no adequate means of assessing the 'efficiency' of the male reproductive system. The measures of male fertility in use today have poor predictive value. One survey of men undergoing elective vasectomy, all of whom had had at least one child, rated 20 per cent of them as infertile (Nelson and Bunge, 1974, p. 503). And studies of semen used in artificial insemination have shown that these measures cannot predict the most successful donors (Friberg and Gemzell, 1977, p. 153). In an editorial in the prestigious journal *Fertility and Sterility* in 1980, two world-renowned urologists (Dubin and Amelar, 1980) pleaded for a more scientific approach to male fertility. And again two years later, another urologist points to the conflicts and confusions created by the enigma of male fertility as numerous authorities 'endeavour to define once and for all the limits of seminal fluid "adequacy"' (Lipshultz, 1982, p. 153). These debates about adequacy centre on reviewing the numerical limits of the same old measures; rarely are the measures themselves challenged. Young points out that:

> By representing variations in numerical forms, the quantitative approach tends to direct our attention away from evaluation of the concepts and variables themselves . . . the investigator becomes concerned with the quantitative presence, absence and variations of the phenomena – at the expense of qualitative and evaluative debates about the different ways of seeing and engaging in events. (Young, 1979, p. 68)

It is the endeavour itself, the attempt to quantify male fertility, which lies at the heart of the problem.

Why is the measurement of male fertility so problematic? I will argue that it is because of the contradiction between defining spermatozoa in terms of individual, independent actors, a temptation found irresistible by science and medicine, and the sheer numbers of sperm found in many different shapes and sizes in a single ejaculate.

The idea that sperm are individual actors responsible for fertilisation can be traced back to Leeuwenhoek, who in the seventeenth century was the first person to see and describe sperm. Then, it was believed that each sperm contained the 'homunculus', meaning little man, that grew to maturity when placed in the womb of the female. From Leeuwenhoek's lifetime 'advances in visualisation were less than dramatic . . . major breakthroughs did not come until the 1950s with the introduction of the electron microscope' (Special Article, 1980, p. 12). Nevertheless, it appears that some of the assumptions arising from Leeuwenhoek's observations inform the measures of male fertility in use today.

Nearly every writer on male fertility indulges in a panegyric on the sperm's qualities, its supposed capacity for independent, purposeful existence. Examples abound, but I have restricted myself to a few which should suffice to illustrate my point. Each sperm consists of a head, that 'nuclear war-head of paternal genes' (Passmore and Robson, 1968, p. 28), which represents the 'most concentrated accumulation of information in the universe' (Macfarlane-Burnett, 1973, p. 54). The head fertilises the egg and is powered by an active tail; 'all else is sacrificed to subserve these two functions' (Passmore and Robson, 1968, p. 28).

> Sperm are all equipped with individual tails that enable them to propel themselves forward. Like salmon, they must swim upstream, first passing through the cervix, then navigating the relatively ample space of the uterus, then finding their way to the small opening of the tubes, only one of which leads to the single egg, and finally swimming against the currents of the hairs in the tube to reach the area of the tube where fertilisation must take place . . . the sperm must travel a distance of approximately three thousand times its own length. This is equivalent to a six foot person swimming three miles upstream. (Harrison, 1979, p. 19)

Sperm are self-motivated to undertake this hazardous journey:

> As cells, spermatozoa are in a class by themselves . . . It is an actively mobile cell, in many ways resembling a free living microorganism, whose only function is to race in the direction where an ovum may be waiting to be fertilized – and to be the first of some 300 million competitors to reach the ovum. (Macfarlane-Burnett, 1973, p. 54)

Not surprisingly, 'the male-producing sperm being lighter and thinner, will enter the albumen faster than the female producers . . . remaining behind are predominantly the female producers plus the less viable males' (Special Article, 1980, p. 17).

What of the ovum? It is unremarkable: a secondary oocyte in an arrested state of meitotic division. (Begley *et al.* 1980, p. 3)

There is no firm evidence to show that the sperm is capable of a self-motivated independent existence; in fact, most of the evidence points to the contrary. 'The function of the [sperm] nucleus is concerned with the future embryo rather than with the spermatozoon itself' (Bishop and Walton, 1956, p. 43). This is confirmed by research carried out for in vitro fertilisation techniques, which reports that:

> Spermatozoa are not directionally oriented during their passage through the vagina, uterus and fallopian tubes – their individual tracts tend to be circular rather than straight and there is no evidence that they can show chemotactic attraction . . . on deposition in the uterus or vagina, the spermatozoa tend to disperse in all directions, rather like gas molecules from a focal point. (Austin, 1974, p. 96)

How do sperm find their way to the ovum? 'General orientation is imposed by the structural or mechanical features of the female organs and the sperm are drawn along the female reproductive tract by the peristaltic motion' (Austin, 1974, p. 96).

It is the early version of sperm as independent actors which has informed the measures of fertility. This version appears to have developed from sperm performance in the laboratory. Ruth Herschberger tells of a physician who in 1939 complained that sperm tests had little to do with fertility. Rather, he complained, sperm were being tested for 'the pleasure of seeing them display maximum motility under artificial conditions' (Herschberger, 1970, p. 68). The performance of sperm in a laboratory, i.e. taken from a sterile plastic jar and placed on a slide for examination under a microscope, may have little to do with their experience in the female reproductive tract.

Sperm may be fun to observe in a laboratory but their performance as individuals has doubtful relevance in terms of predicting fertility. Individual sperm are judged in terms of their morphology (that is, their appearance) and in terms of their motility (their ability to actively progress or wriggle about). Behind these measures lies the assumption that only a nicely-shaped, active and purposeful sperm can fertilise an egg.

How are the nicely-shaped sperm selected from the others? Human sperm is unique in that unlike all other species, it shows marked differences in size and shape in an ejaculate and between men. Why this occurs in man only, the origin of this discrepancy and its significance in terms of fertility are all as yet unexplained. This variability however, presents enormous problems in terms of reliability of measurement. One researcher sent microphotographs of 500 human sperm to 47 experts and received widely differing opinions of 50 per cent of the specimens. He concluded that 'sperm morphology is very often a case of beauty in the eye of the beholder' (Freund,1966). Hence, we find statements in textbooks such as 'Moench [the pioneer of work on sperm morphology] considers very long, tapering and narrow sperm heads of especially sinister import' (Payling Wright and Symmers, 1966, p. 396).

The significance of motility in individual sperm is unclear especially once it is accepted that sperm cannot swim. Furthermore, 'although good quality semen samples contain vigorously motile spermatozoa, motility in itself may be regarded as a separate entity from the mechanism of fertilisation' (Mann, 1977, p. 431). It is generally accepted that not all motile sperm are fertile, nevertheless it is assumed that only a motile sperm is capable of fertilisation.

> Now, impossibilities are in the nature of the case difficult to demonstrate, and in science the history of such claims is an inglorious one: over and over what one period was convinced just couldn't be done was subsequently accomplished – though to be sure, usually in a rather different form than was originally conceived. (Kaplan, 1964, p. 212)

This surely must apply to male fertility and the mechanism of fertilisation; and just because no-one has yet observed an immotile sperm fertilise an ovum, that does not mean that all immotile sperm are incapable of so doing.

Once the panegyric on individual sperm has been delivered, male fertility is discussed in terms of the overall quality of semen. However, the qualities of sperm as individuals have informed the measures of male fertility used today: sperm numbers, sperm morphology and sperm motility. The last two, morphology and motility, are now expressed as proportionate qualities of the total ejaculate. A 'normal' semen sample has a sperm count of 200 million, 60 per cent of which are morphologically nicely-shaped and 60 per cent of which are actively motile. These overall measures of semen are then said to correlate with fertility and not the presence of a few able-bodied sperm.

Focusing on sperm as individual actors in fertilisation leads to confusion about the function of the vast numbers expended in a single ejaculate. This confusion is demonstrated by the frequent revisions downward of the number of sperm compatible with fertility; the cut-off point has been lowered from 80 million to 40 million, still a vast number. Furthermore, this focus impedes any investigation into the molecular properties of sperm.

> The structural analysis of spermatozoon has probably been carried further than has that of any other differentiated cell type, yet the essential molecular mechanisms of motility . . . still eludes us. (Passmore and Robson, 1968, p. 396)

Conceptualising semen as an aggregate of individual sperm may lead to what Galtung calls the 'fallacy of the wrong level'. This fallacy:

> consists not in making inferences from one level of analysis to another, but in making direct translation of properties or relations from one level to another, i.e. making too simple inferences. The fallacy can be committed working downwards, by projecting from groups or categories to individuals, or upwards, by projecting from individuals to higher units'. (Galtung, 1967, p. 45)

Morphology and motility may be measures of the fitness of individual sperm, but it does not follow that these same measures hold for semen as a whole. 'It is not possible to predict from the properties of elementary components which of all possible complex structures will in fact arise' (Scazzocchio, 1982, p. 80). The enigma of male fertility remains because, since Leeuwenhoek, medicine has failed to conceptualise measures of fertility which engage with semen as anything other than an aggregate of 200 million individual, competing actors.

The fact that the mechanism of male fertility is not clearly understood can in part explain the absence of non-mechanical means of contraception for controlling male fertility. Also it is evident that treatment for male fertility is not based upon clearly understood principles, but on empirical treatment, such as vitamins and hormones, which are used on a 'try it and see' basis and acknowledged to be ineffective (Hudson *et al.* 1980, p. 106).

Fertility in men is further distinguished from that in women because it does end discretely, i.e. men do not go through a menopause. One consequence of this is the belief that fertility in men persists often into old age. Clearly, no complicated laboratory investigations into a woman's fertility are needed after the menopause. But what proof is there that 'although interest and activity decline with advancing years, physically healthy men can remain fertile in the eighth or ninth decade'? (Smith, 1978, p. 33)

Three factors undermine such claims. Firstly, as Ruth Herschberger points out, 'no-one knows to what extent the man of fifty is sterile; there have been no surveys which can categorically prove fertility one way or another' (Herschberger, 1970, p. 56). And because sterility and impotence are so often confused in men, a man's fertility is often tested merely by self-reports of erection and ejaculation. Secondly, the measures of male fertility in use are poor predictors of fertility; only fatherhood is sufficient. So whilst spermatogenesis may indeed persist, few men have their fertility status tested in later life. The scientific method itself encourages a search for a significant difference, for falsification of a null hypothesis. Hence, when an elderly man becomes a father, this is taken as proof of potential fertility in all elderly men rather than as a unique, freak event which needs to be explained away. Lastly, there is medical evidence that the male reproductive organs, in fact, atrophy with age, although the significance of this in terms of fertility cannot be stated. The few morphological studies of testes in elderly men show evidence of reduced spermatogenesis. 'Changes in hormone levels and testis morphology are correlated with an increasing incidence of the clinical features of hypogonadism (decreased functional activity of the testes) as senescence approaches – testicular atrophy, loss of body hair and reduced sexual function' (Hudson and Burger, 1979, p. 91). Ruth Herschberger sums up the issue as follows: 'only because sterility and impotence are so often confused has it seemed important to men that their fertility remain unquestioned into the grave' (Herschberger, 1970, p. 61).

Susan Sontag points out that:

> Ageing is much more a social judgement than a biological eventuality . . . This society allows men to have a much more affirmative relation to their bodies than women have. Men are 'at home' in their bodies whether they treat them casually or aggressively. A man's body is described as a strong body . . . Consequently, men rarely panic about ageing in the way women often do. (Sontag, 1978, p. 76)

The biological basis of this social judgement is questionable; we must look to the social construction of medical knowledge for its persistence.

Conclusion

This chapter presents a first step towards a feminist analysis of the medical approach to *both* men's and women's reproductive health. As such it represents a departure from previous feminist analyses which traditionally have examined women's reproductive health in isolation from men's. This approach is in many ways inevitable, given the visibility of women as consumers of medicine. But I would argue that a feminist analysis which focuses on women alone is in danger of reproducing and reinforcing the very medical definitions it sets out to challenge.

Including men alongside women in our analysis changes the nature of the debate. It enables us to see the pressure to define women's health largely in terms of reproductive health. We can now ask how important is reproduction in terms of women's health. As this chapter demonstrates, medicine can make disease both visible and invisible. Feminists have overlooked other health issues relevant to women in the struggle over definitions of reproductive health. Reproduction is only one of our body's systems and should be placed in a context for a clearer understanding of women's health needs.

Reproduction is nonetheless unique in that it is the only bodily function not essential for the maintenance of an individual's survival; rather, as de Beauvoir (1972) points out, it is concerned with the furtherance of the human species and as such carries meaning and significance different from say digestion or respiration. Because it is the only bodily function that is different in men and women, it lies at the heart of debates about gender. This chapter has demonstrated that the very language and terms of the debate are themselves gendered.

Acknowledgement
I would like to thank Anne Woollett for reading numerous versions of this paper.

4 The Medical Construction of the Contraceptive Career

Hilary Thomas

In Britain during the twentieth century there have been major changes in the use of contraception (e.g. Woolf, 1971; Bone, 1973, 1978; Langford, 1976; Dunnell, 1979). The increase in use of methods of contraception by women has been accompanied by a growing involvement on the part of the medical profession. Most female methods are deemed to require medical intervention: the oral and injectable contraceptives require prescription; the intra-uterine contraceptive device (IUCD), the diaphragm and the cervical cap must be fitted; the various techniques used to establish the rhythm method require advice. Provision of these methods has become largely the province of medical personnel rather than, for example, nurses or midwives, trained lay people, or women themselves.[1]

The development of family planning services has been described elsewhere (Leathard, 1980). The general attitudes to fertility control held by general practitioners, gynaecologists and surgeons have been explored by Aitken-Swan (1977). A growing volume of literature presents women's views of different methods and the services which provide them (e.g. Phillips and Rakusen, 1979; Mackeith, 1978). Other studies have drawn attention to differential access to contraception amongst women (Christopher, 1980), and one recent study has pointed to the paucity of information and advice available to men (Birth Control Trust, 1984).

This chapter does not attempt to address the issues raised in existing studies of contraception. It takes the form of a review of the literature written by doctors for members of their profession, examines in more detail the medical view of the function of contraception and the factors which constitute the medical construction of the contraceptive needs of their patients. Studies in other areas of reproduction have indicated that decisions made by doctors are influenced not only by the state of medical knowledge of reproduction but also by their perceptions of social and cultural norms (Macintyre, 1976; Fisher, 1984). Articles and letters which have appeared in the *British Medical*

Journal (BMJ) during the past thirty years provide an insight into the different ways contraception has been viewed by the medical profession. In addition, the variety of contraceptive methods available has lead to the publication of a number of books which are intended to assist chiefly general practitioners with their advice and choice of methods for patients. For example the cover of *Practical Contraception* (Ramaswamy and Smith, 1976) states,

> This extremely practical book is written for the busy practising doctor. It sets out a strategy of contraception, in which advice is given on the selection of the best forms of fertility control for an individual patient, on the problems which may be encountered with the various forms of contraception, and on related conditions such as the menopause, psychosexual disorders and sexually transmitted diseases.

These books contain information about different methods of contraception and the types of patients for whom they are considered suitable. Suitability is based on both medical and social factors, that is, there are medical views of social factors which are considered to have a bearing on the choice of contraceptive method, in addition to the assessment of medical indications. The BMJ, the journal which GPs are most likely to read, also contains information about choice of method.

This critical view of the literature examines the selection of social factors and the reasons why they are considered to be relevant to the choice of contraceptive method. Several authors suggest that the contraceptive needs of individuals change during the reproductive lifetime, suggesting that different stages in the contraceptive history can be identified (BMJ Leading Article, 1976; Ramaswamy and Smith, 1976; International Planned Parenthood Federation, 1980). This chapter examines the identification of these different stages and concludes that this comprises the medical construction of a contraceptive career. In order to examine these issues this chapter raises the following questions. What is the function of contraception and what is it seen as preventing? What are the criteria by which methods are chosen for patients? What are the stages in the reproductive life-cycle which the medical profession assumes are associated with changing contraceptive needs?

The function of contraception

Examination of the BMJ during the last 30 years with respect to contraception and family planning, reveals that the attitudes of the medical profession to contraception and family planning have undergone many changes. At any one time it is difficult to identify single universally held opinions. The dissenting voice is usually to be heard – chiefly in the correspondence columns but sometimes in 'Personal View' or in an article elsewhere. Analysis of the views expressed requires more lengthy treatment than is possible in this chapter, but it is possible to identify some of the major functions of contraception as conceptualised by the medical profession. In addition to preventing pregnancy, contraception has been seen to prevent the following: danger to health from pregnancy or fear of pregnancy (Medical Women's Federation, 1952); grand multiparity, i.e. having 'too many' children (Sadler, 1952b; BMJ Leading Article, 1972); having births too closely spaced (Pyke, 1952; Nicolas and Nicolas, 1972); illegitimacy (Gifford *et al.* 1971); abortion (Gifford *et al.* 1971; BMJ Leading Article, 1973); overpopulation (BMJ Leading Article, 1972); and the costs to the community of unwanted or undesirable pregnancies (Wilson, 1971).

Before considering each of these functions in turn I shall outline briefly the topics of discussion about contraception which have occurred in the BMJ over the last thirty years. In the early 1950s discussion was mainly confined to whether or not married women should be able to obtain contraceptive advice and supplies from doctors for non-medical reasons, that is for reasons other than avoiding likely danger from pregnancy. Questions from doctors about contraceptive methods were restricted to diaphragms, spermicides and the use of the safe period. In 1958 in response to a question about the latest information on oral contraception, the BMJ expert wrote:

> It is encouraging that a good deal of high quality research into the problem of devising the ideal contraceptive is now being undertaken by first-class investigators, and though 'the pill' in its ideal form is probably still a long way off optimism would appear to be not unwarranted. (BMJ, 1958, p. 1116)

From then on the BMJ contains many articles about particular varieties of pill and their effectiveness. Side effects of the pill and contra-indications for those who ought not to be prescribed it became major themes after the mid 1960s. There is a brief correspondence early in the 1960s in which the wisdom of giving healthy women systemic drugs is questioned, and in which various doctors suggest that the duty of the doctor should be confined to treating the sick. The IUCD joins the pill as a leading method in the late 1960s. In the early 1970s three main issues are discussed: implications of the large number of abortions performed each year as a result of the 1967 Abortion Act; the role of doctors in population control; and the provision of contraception to the unmarried. In the mid 1970s there is concern following the reorganisation of the National Health Service in 1974 and the implications for provision of services, with payment to GPs for *their* family planning services, and the removal of prescription charges for contraceptives. After the mid 1970s the number of technical articles, letters and questions about contraception declines quite rapidly. Reflecting this decline, a leading article in 1979 is headed with the question 'Tomorrow's contraceptive: yesterday's problem?' (BMJ Leading Article, 1979).

Each of the functions of contraception listed earlier has been incorporated into the current view of contraception held by the medical profession, but each became seen as important at a different time. Each function will be discussed in chronological order.

Spacing and limiting numbers

During the early 1950s discussion centred on the advisability of allowing married women access to birth control for medical *and* for family spacing reasons. In 1952 a brisk correspondence resulted from a recommendation by the Family Planning Committee of the Medical Women's Federation:

> We recommend that advice on family planning should be available to women who ask for it on medical grounds, *and also to women who ask for it for the purpose of family spacing*. (Medical Women's Federation, 1952, p. 596)

In reply, Dr Sadler suggested that whilst medical grounds were acceptable, family spacing was likely to have unfortunate consequences, in particular a fall in the birth rate,

> Let us have a Family Planning Association by all means – but let it be an association whose avowed aim is to *help mothers overcome the social factors which tend to make them wish to limit their families*. (Sadler, 1952a, p. 868)

She suggested that the voluntary assistants at FPA clinics would be better occupied with voluntary housework for hard-pressed mothers. Dr Joan Malleson replied,

> I think if Dr Sadler would join a Family Planning Association clinic for an afternoon she would find grateful patients assuring her that their contraceptive security has done more to help the stability of family life than a whole stream of friendly enthusiasts coming to assist with their housework could ever do. (Malleson, 1952, p. 970)

Dr Sadler then suggested that, although *initially* unwanted, many mothers continued with a pregnancy which eventually lead to the birth of a much loved member of the family, capable of giving support to parents in their old age. Thus, she argued, the medical profession should take the long-term view and not the emotional one,

> *Our* duty must lie in giving advice, if asked, *on medical grounds only* (one took it that multiparity of four or five children could be reasonably classified as 'medical grounds'). Beyond this we have no responsibility. (Sadler, 1952b, p. 1132)

Margaret Pyke, Honorary Secretary to the Family Planning Association (FPA) took up the theme of large families:

> By all means let us do our best to create an atmosphere, and indeed a world in which large families will be welcome and well-fed, but we shall never get anywhere near either unless families are both spaced and limited. (Pyke, 1952, p. 1028)

Other correspondents suggested that women wished to limit their families for frivolous, materialistic reasons (e.g. Waddy, 1952). Letters challenging this view 'defended' women on the basis that most seemed to *want* a large family but felt they could only make adequate provision for a limited number of children (Jones, 1952).

Throughout this correspondence the major theme is the grounds on which women 'deserve' access to contraceptive advice and supplies. It is only in their role as mothers that women can call on the medical profession for assistance, unless medical necessity prevails. What women might choose for themselves in terms of the number and frequency of births on any other grounds than good motherhood is not considered. What is at issue in the above correspondence is what constitutes good mothering.

It appears that even by the early 1970s, when the debate had moved to issues such as the provision of services for the unmarried and the doctor's role in population control, provision for those who wished to space and limit their families or those who had been advised to do so, was inadequate:

> It has long been one of the axioms of obstetrics that mothers should have at least two-year gaps between the births of their babies, but how little advice has been given over the years to enable them to achieve this. (Nicolas and Nicolas, 1972, p. 52)

It seems clear that the medical necessity for spacing and limiting the number of births in the family had been established. Grand multiparity was the target of several points in letters and Leading Articles. The word 'feckless' frequently appears, suggesting, perhaps, that those who have large families are necessarily 'feckless'. Certainly the large, planned family is rarely mentioned (Oldershaw, 1975).

> Family doctors will have to seek out the feckless and problem

families in their practice and take contraception to them. (BMJ Leading Article, 1972, p. 391)

However it would not be until contraceptive provision was made available within the NHS that doctors would,

> . . . feel free to urge feckless, fecund multigravidae to agree to some sort of long-term defence against repeated pregnancy. (BMJ Leading Article, 1972, p. 391)

Illegitimacy, abortion and unwanted pregnancy

If contraception was viewed as controlling the number of children and the spacing of births within the family, it was also intended that its use could emphasise marriage as the proper locus of reproduction. Contraception could prevent illegitimacy (Gifford *et al.* 1971). The passing of the 1967 Abortion Act resulted in an increasing number of pregnancies being terminated. There was considerable debate in medical circles concerning doctors' legal ability to authorise termination whilst being unable to prescribe free contraception within the NHS unless for strictly medical reasons. Contraception became seen as a way of preventing abortion; in particular it could prevent the *demand* for abortion which some doctors felt had resulted in gynaecologists being reduced to technicians, a view which disregarded the gynaecologists' power to withhold consent to a termination (Gifford *et al.* 1971). Contraception could also reduce the number of unwanted pregnancies, evidenced by the number of abortions each year.

The use of the term 'unwanted pregnancy' in this literature requires critical attention. Abortion figures are usually cited to indicate the number of unwanted pregnancies but this can be regarded as a conservative indication. Abortion figures only represent those unwanted pregnancies which the medical profession has agreed to terminate. It does not include those whose applications were rejected nor those who did not even approach their doctor because, for example, they believed that an application would be turned down. It is known that abortion is more easily obtained by single than by married women on social grounds. A married woman with no or few children is less likely to be treated sympathetically. This distinction arises from the belief that single women are less likely to be in an appropriate social and financial position to raise a child. Marriage as the proper locus of reproduction is supported by this interpretation of the 1967 Act. Thus when the medical profession indicates that contraception can be used to prevent unwanted pregnancies, its primary concern is with undesirability as defined by the medical profession, rather than with unwantedness as defined by the pregnant woman. As Macintyre has noted, the medical profession frequently fails to distinguish between unplanned, unwanted and undesirable pregnancies (Macintyre, 1975).

In a leading article entitled 'Abortion or Contraception?' in 1971 the BMJ argued that doctors should be free to prescribe contraception on social grounds rather than acceding to abortion on demand, and that they should encourage the attitude that unless a child is wanted, sexual intercourse without contraception be regarded as,

> . . . an act of selfish irresponsibility . . . Effective contraception is available, and there should be no excuse for unintentional pregnancies. (BMJ Leading Article 1971, p. 261)

Two correspondents wrote to support the principle of contraception available on the NHS, but to disagree with other points. Malcolm Potts suggested that figures for abortion might rise even if contraceptive use increased, since it was not true to say that this was an age of 'effective contraception'; consistent use of recommended methods over a fertile life-time could lead to disappointing results (Potts, 1971). The head of the Student Health Service at Sheffield University, Dr Gifford, wrote,

> Free contraception cannot remove overnight all the social and psychological factors that lead to unwanted pregnancy. (Gifford, 1971, p. 534)

Overpopulation and the cost to the community

Overpopulation and the doctor's role in helping to overcome this provided a major theme for correspondence in 1972. Whilst some correspondents felt it was a doctor's duty to consider also the well-being of the community, others suggested that the exclusive responsibility was to the patient. The subject of morality was raised in connection with population control:

> Widespread publicity on methods of population control in the absence of strong motivations towards continent family living could be regarded as a move directed intentionally against marriage. (Mackay, 1972, p. 244)

It was suggested that the costs of services could be offset against the savings made: contraception prevented waste. In describing the Domiciliary Family Planning Service in Glasgow, Elizabeth Wilson commented,

> Although the service is expensive in professional time, the overall saving in costs to the community by the prevention of unwanted pregnancies in socially inadequate families fully justifies the scheme. (Wilson, 1971, p. 731)

Debate about who should be allowed access to contraceptive services lessened during the late 1970s, with the exception of the subject of provision for under-16 year olds. A leading article in 1973 reflected this:

> The general approval amongst doctors for the principle of NHS contraception reflects the changes in the profession's attitudes to sexual medicine in recent years. Discussion has moved away from theorising about morals and has concentrated on the practical problems of reducing the numbers of unwanted pregnancies . . . (BMJ Leading Article, 1973, p. 130)

This chapter so far has shown that contraception has been seen to prevent several different social phenomena. Each of the categories discussed above are considered to be functions of contraception. Latterly there *appears* to be more freedom to choose in matters of reproduction. However it is obviously debatable whether there is in fact free choice in whether or not women have children and how many they have. Through an examination of what contraception is considered to prevent, it has been shown that use of contraception allows for the confining of procreation to marriage. Spacing and limiting of births not only protects maternal health but also allows for 'better' mothering and hence for more stable families. Contraceptive services for the unmarried have been established to prevent illegitimacy and abortion rather than to promote sexual freedom.

The criteria for choice

In this chapter the term 'choice' is used to describe choice by doctors of methods suitable for patients. However it is important to note that, particularly, feminists are pressing for informed choice (e.g. Rakusen, 1981, 1982). Most authors of books concerning contraception written for doctors point to the importance of the method being acceptable to the patient. Some suggest that the doctor should describe all methods with their advantages and limitations and allow the patient to choose the eventual method once medical contra-indications have been established (e.g. Pollock, 1966; International Planned Parenthood Federation, 1980). However the descriptions of methods and situations in which they might be applicable indicate that the ideas which the medical profession has about appropriate methods are based on medical *and* social factors. It is likely, therefore, that preconceived notions of the matching of patients and methods will influence the doctor when giving contraceptive care and may lead to the more frequent recommendation of some methods rather than others. The criteria for choice of method which are regularly discussed in the literature can be grouped under five main headings: male or female methods; physiological factors; the need to prevent pregnancy; motivation of the patient to use and continue to use the method; and sexual behaviour and sexual relationships.

Male or female methods

Most methods are for women's use and most contraceptive users are women. The main reversible male method, the sheath, does not require medical supervision. The typical contraceptive patient, as constructed in the literature, is a woman, though sometimes 'the patient' is a couple. Men as individuals are not generally thought to be in need of advice or information about contraception. However, this view is challenged by Oldershaw:

> It is also arguable that as the female is the one at risk from unwanted pregnancy and abortion, the contraceptive effort should be directed at her rather than at the male. Nonetheless, the family doctor should indicate his willingness to provide contraception to the adolescent males. In my experience they rarely come back to me for advice themselves, but occasionally send, and may even bring, their girl friends along. (Oldershaw, 1975, p. 37)

General practitioners cannot prescribe supplies of sheaths under the NHS, though supplies are freely available from clinics. The main reason appears to be that the method does not require medical intervention for use and as such is outside the province of the GP. Indeed there was vigorous opposition to the idea that GPs might prescribe sheaths:

> It is surely the last straw if the government intends to insult us by filling our surgeries with a lot of louts queuing up for the issue of condoms. (Phillips, 1973, p. 782)

Perhaps because the sheath does not require medical prescription or supervision, the literature tends to emphasise its use rather less than other methods such as the pill, IUCD, and diaphragm. The sheath appears as a method whose use should not be discouraged in those couples for whom it is already a satisfactory method (Peel and Potts, 1971; Oldershaw, 1975). Its use is not actively encouraged except in particular situations, for example, Peel and Potts (1971) suggest that it is a useful method for those couples for whom intercourse is sporadic and unpredictable, or for those couples who wish to share the responsibility for contraception. It is noteworthy that 'sharing responsibility' is presented as a strategy of contraception which comes from the couple themselves: it is not implied that doctors should suggest this to couples.

The business of contraceptive care by the medical profession is presented as essentially the work of prescription or fitting of appliances rather than provision of information. As such the services are directed towards the users of methods rather than participants in heterosexual activity. Barnes states,

> Counselling for family planning will generally consist of an interview with the woman. Sometimes a man may come for advice but this is unusual. Such advice would consist of advice on how most safely to use the condom, with, in suitable situations, a discussion of vasectomy. (Barnes, 1976, p. 9)

This view implies that women and men are not instructed in the use of each other's method or how an individual can best give support to a partner using a particular method. It would be interesting to know how many consultations for contraceptive care do contain information and advice about *all* methods of contraception. Many people know of the sheath as a method, but as contraception is now seen by many as a subject requiring medical advice, failure to discuss the sheath might lead to its removal from a list of methods considered by the individual or couple. A tendency on the part of the medical profession not to discuss male methods of contraception reinforces the idea that contraception is a woman's responsibility.

Physiological factors

The age of the female patient is taken to be an indication of her fertility – thus a woman in her late thirties or older is presumed to be less fertile and therefore the risk of pregnancy is presumed to be less. As the pill, which has the greatest degree of ability to prevent pregnancy other than sterilisation, is not recommended for older women, another method with a higher risk of failure is often considered to be sufficiently reliable. Very young women whose menstruation shows signs of anovulatory cycles are often advised not to take the pill until ovulation has been established. This is in order to prevent infertility in later years, since if ovulation has not been properly established before its suppression with oral contraception it may be difficult to establish it at a later date. The *maintenance* of potential fertility is also a criterion for choice of method, for example the IUCD is sometimes not recommended for nulliparous women in case infection leads to sterility, amongst other reasons. The need to maintain potential fertility is usually assumed rather than discussed with the patient. Women who have been pregnant may find the IUCD more acceptable than those who have not, though a group of devices has been designed with the constraints of the nulliparous patient in mind, for example, the copper 7. If a woman is breast feeding the combined oral contraceptive may be contra-indicated because the hormones contained in the pill might affect lactation.

In addition to the above features individuals may have particular conditions which contra-indicate use of particular methods. This is particularly so with systemic methods such as the pill.

The need to prevent pregnancy

One of the most important factors to be considered when assessing methods of contraception is their ability to prevent pregnancy. However it is not the only factor, nor for some people is it the most important, as this literature seems to suggest. Whilst it is probable that an individual or couple who wish to avoid pregnancy would want to choose the most reliable method, other considerations such as side effects and aesthetic acceptability will also be considered. Within the literature there are references to situations in which the need to prevent pregnancy outweighs other factors, according to the judgement of these authors. Those who are seen by the medical profession to most need to prevent pregnancy include the young, the single, those whose health would be at risk from pregnancy, and those who have completed child-bearing.

Peel and Potts (1971) make clear the association between the need to prevent pregnancy in single women, and the consequent need to use the safest method of contraception, the pill:

> It is in the clear interest of both society and the individual to make contraceptive advice available to the unmarried as well as the married. It does not lead to promiscuity, but it may prevent some unwanted pregnancies and enable some more mature and responsible marriages to take place . . . It is important to use the most effective and acceptable method and oral contraceptives are nearly always the first choice. (Peel and Potts, 1971, p. 234)

Similarly in a chapter entitled 'Advice to the young and single', Ramaswamy and Smith say,

> In effect, then, the choice of first contraceptive for teenage girls is restricted to the pill or an IUD. Most girls can be persuaded to start oral contraception – it seems an adult, sophisticated thing to do – and the virtual guarantee of protection from pregnancy is a great advantage. (Ramaswamy and Smith, 1976, p. 11)

For those who have completed childbearing and who do not wish to maintain their potential fertility, sterilisation of one or other partner is often suggested as an alternative (Barnes, 1976).

The need to avoid pregnancy is not thought to be so great in those who are spacing pregnancies:

> The young woman whose main concern is the spacing of her family presents rather different needs for contraceptive advice

> than the teenager whose main concern is the avoidance of pregnancy. (Ramaswamy and Smith, 1976, p. 4)

It is ironic that spacing pregnancies should be regarded as requiring a relatively less efficient method of contraception. One of the most important functions of contraception in the 1950s was precisely that women might be able to space their pregnancies and this was deemed to be good medical advice. It could be argued that a woman who is spacing births should use the most effective method during this period of her life since the medical perception of her situation might be less sympathetic and an application for abortion be more difficult to negotiate.

By implication the woman who is spacing births could consider other factors:

> . . . she may be one of the many women who stop taking the pill in order to have their first child and only then realise how much better they feel when freed of the influence of hormonal contraception. These two changes, a lowered tolerance of the side effects of hormonal contraception and less emphasis on the need to prevent pregnancy, may tip the balance in favour of an intrauterine device. (Ramaswamy and Smith, 1976, p. 4)

Oldershaw says that in all cases,

> The method chosen should therefore be the most effective method that the patient finds acceptable. (Oldershaw, 1975, p. 264)

It seems, however, that the young, single, nulliparous might be *encouraged* to tolerate, for example, side effects from the pill and that 'acceptability' might be a matter of negotiation between patient and doctor, not a matter of individual feeling. In the eyes of the medical profession, the need to avoid pregnancy varies with the marital and reproductive status rather than the aspirations of the individual.

Motivation

There is much discussion about assessment of the motivation of the patient to use contraception, and to continue to use particular methods. In this literature motivation is a blanket term, a word used simply to describe whether or not a woman seems likely to use the contraceptive method in question. It is *not* an explanatory term, in that it does not explain why women do or do not use contraception at various times. The use of the term motivation in this sense seems to *proscribe* adequate explanations of why people do or do not use contraception.

Motivation, or the supposed lack of it, is particularly associated with using the IUCD, injectable contraceptives and sterilisation, methods considered suitable for 'feckless' women. An example of the type of comment which appears frequently is found in an article in the BMJ,

> The loop or coil is the method of choice for the unmotivated patient, giving the maximum protection with the minimum of effort. (Law, 1971, p. 444)

Barnes (1976) suggests that the woman's motivation and success or failure with past methods will help the doctor in advising on a method:

> Women can be roughly divided into two main categories: those who can be safely relied on to adhere to a method, such as the contraceptive pill or a diaphragm, that they must use themselves; and those for whom the method advised must not depend on them as, for example, the intrauterine device, sterilisation or possibly an injectable contraceptive. (Barnes, 1976, p. 11)

The term 'feckless' is frequently used. Oldershaw gives a description of this term,

> 'Feckless females' is a generic term used to cover the type of women all GPs know very well. Of inadequate personality, low intelligence and prone to anxiety, they are bound to miss Pills, or stop taking them without seeking medical advice. Side effects can be guaranteed to be severe and multitudinous. Recurrent unwanted pregnancies and pitiful pleas for abortion will result. (Oldershaw, 1975, p. 265)

Oldershaw also discusses what he feels to be the proper concern of the medical practitioner with the efficiency of contraception used by women after abortion:

> In such circumstances it seems to be that the patient often needs protection, not only against pregnancy, but also against herself. To insist on the use of a reliable, reversible method of contraception after abortion, seems to me reasonable, and if a patient of mine would not agree to use a method, I would question my estimate of her need for abortion. To insist that the method used is one which the patient cannot fail to use seems a logical extension. (Oldershaw, 1975, p. 263)

There seems little room in this situation for the woman's definition of either her need for abortion or her requirements of future contraception.

The provision of care to women from ethnic minorities is rarely mentioned apart from occasional references to cultural difficulties for some women with side effects of methods such as the IUCD (e.g. Oldershaw, 1975, p. 258). However concepts of family planning and spacing may be quite inappropriate for women from different cultures which have different ideas and beliefs about family size and the meaning of children.

Sexual behaviour and sexual relationships

The authors of this literature are aware of some of the problems of using contraception in the context of a sexual relationship. However these are mostly in one direction. Much is made of implications of different types of sexual relationship for the choice of contraceptive method but there is little or no reference to the effect of different contraceptive methods, once chosen, on the developing relationship. Most of the texts contain a section or chapter devoted to sexual problems, but such problems are usually discussed independently of contraception. References to spontaneity and aesthetics are the closest that most texts come to discussing the effect of different methods on sexual behaviour.

In discussing the implications of what the medical profession perceives as different sexual relationships perhaps requiring different methods of contraception, the pre-existence of a relationship is always assumed. What most authors fail to take into account is that using, or discussing, methods once a relationship is established is very different from using, or preparing to use, methods in the very early stages of the relationship, i.e. during the time of the establishment of the relationship and before the instance of first intercourse. It has been suggested that the sheath be given wider publicity in an effort to make it more acceptable to younger age groups (Cossey, 1979). However, since GPs do not prescribe the method and family planning clinics are directed mainly towards women there would appear to be difficulties with this idea. A recent project has begun to investigate the potential for involving pharmacists in the campaign to make contraception more widely available (Meredith, 1982). One of the methods of contraception currently under experiment, in fact an old idea recycled, is the use of the vaginal sponge containing spermicide. This can be inserted several hours before intercourse. It is made in one size and so does not require fitting by a trained person. If the method were to be marketed, women would have available a method which they could obtain in similar ways to that of the sheath, e.g. pharmacists, slot machines, etc.

Assuming the existence of the heterosexual relationship, the literature does make appeal to different 'stages' in a relationship. This is particularly evident in discussion of the relative merits and limitations of coitus-independent and coitus-dependent methods. Young couples in particular are thought to benefit from the coitus-independent aspect of the pill which,

> . . . is of particular value when they have no previous sexual experience. Oral contraception permits them fully spontaneous sexual expression at all times. (IPPF, 1980, p. 53)

Opinion is divided about the acceptability of mechanical methods, such as the diaphragm, later on in a relationship in which coitus-independent methods have been used. On the one level Ramaswamy and Smith argue that a barrier method may become more acceptable:

> . . . once a couple have established a satisfactory sexual relationship they are more likely to tolerate the lack of spontaneity inevitable when a diaphragm or condom is used. (Ramaswamy and Smith, 1976, p. 4)

However Guillebaud (1975) has argued that use of oral contraception for many years 'spoils' women and leads to poor motivation to use a diaphragm. Elsewhere the 'well-adjusted' woman is thought to be able to learn to use the diaphragm in such a way that the 'natural spontaneity' of the relationship is not spoiled. Thus Oldershaw:

> Insertion immediately before intercourse is contraceptively satisfactory, but the wife who says to her husband, 'Hold everything, while I find my cap' is liable to find his ardour dissipated on her return. Even worse, he may verbally apostrophize the thing, and press on regardless. Hence the wise wife should adopt the motto of the Boy Scouts and insert the diaphragm routinely before going to bed. (Oldershaw, 1975, p. 62)

It would seem from this quotation that ideas about 'natural spontaneity' are to be equated with the constant sexual availability of women: women must be in a constant state of preparation for the spontaneous. Or as Bradbury expressed it in quite another context,

> . . . if you want to have something that's genuinely unstructured, you have to plan it carefully. (Bradbury, 1977, p. 7)

There is a conflict between the ideas that mechanical methods 'inevitably' lead to loss of spontaneity and those which imply that if only women would learn to use the diaphragm 'properly' spontaneity could be retained. 'Proper' use of the diaphragm implies either that women must always be ready to supplement the spermicide by the use of pessaries or that there is an implicit structure to the sexual behaviour, e.g. that sex occurs at night. Discovering the hidden 'structure of spontaneity' is assumed to be the woman's task. There is no discussion in the literature of how couples could be encouraged to share in the development of a pattern of sexual and contraceptive behaviour.

The context of contraceptive care is seen as an ideal time for the doctor to encourage discussion of any sexual problems. Pollock (1966) suggests that some patients blame methods of contraception for what might be an 'underlying' sexual problem:

> There are patients whose request for oral contraceptives covers some sexual problem, some blame mechanical methods for their difficulties with intercourse and think the pill will solve their problems. Although this may be so in some cases, the doctor should learn to recognise these patients and make his approach one which will enable them to accept help for their marital problems. This does not mean that oral contraceptives should be refused in these cases, but simply that the doctor and the patient should recognise any underlying difficulties. (Pollock, 1966, p. 5)

Coital frequency is a subject which occurs, especially in discussion of the sheath. There is general agreement that for women for whom intercourse occurs infrequently methods such as the pill and IUCD are inappropriate.

> To take the Pill every night or wear an IUD, with the possible side-effects of both, when one's consort is a seaman or with the Army in Northern Ireland, is plainly carrying contraception too far. (Oldershaw, 1975, p. 67)

In this situation in which a relationship is established, it might well be the case that a couple, whilst resigned to infrequent reunions, would place a premium on spontaneity and a high coital frequency when together. There is little mention of the reality of the life of a woman who has no single established relationship and who has sporadic intercourse. Whilst she may agree or disagree with Oldershaw's assessment that infrequent intercourse is not worth the risk of side effects from the pill or IUD, she still needs contraceptive protection and is not able to predict when she may need this, compared with the partner of the seaman or soldier whose tours of duty are known in advance. A woman in this situation is caught between needing infrequent protection and yet perhaps needing a method which she can use herself and which is also coitus-independent, thus obviating the need to discuss the contraception with the potential partner.

Stages in the reproductive life cycle and contraceptive needs

In 1958 the BMJ heralded research into oral contraception as promising to produce 'the ideal contraceptive' (BMJ, 1958). By 1976 the optimism had waned, somewhat:

> There is no ideal contraceptive. Every woman leading an active sexual life necessarily has to incur the risks of her chosen contraceptive's particular shortcomings and of an unplanned pregnancy should the method let her down. (BMJ Leading Article, 1976, p. 1405)

It had become clear that a range of contraceptive methods would have to be considered by doctors when prescribing for patients. In writing handbooks for busy GPs and in describing the suitability of the various methods in journals, the medical profession has begun to delineate grounds on which patient and method might be matched. The grounds extend well beyond the confines of 'objective medical factors'. Different types of patient and of the situation of the patient have been devised. This has lead to the identification of different stages in lifecycle – the reproductive lifecycle – and of the contraceptive needs which are thought to be associated with each stage (e.g. Ramaswamy and Smith, 1976). These stages are: a sexually active period before childbearing, including perhaps before marriage; a period of childbearing during which pregnancies are spaced; and the period of fertile years after the desired number of children have been born. Women's contraceptive needs are thought to vary over the reproductive lifecycle. For example:

> During her reproductive lifetime she is likely to have varying needs of contraception; the relevant factors include the permanence or otherwise of her sexual relationship, her own career, her desire for children, and whether she wishes to retain her potential for reproduction. (BMJ Leading Article, 1976, p. 1406)

> No one contraceptive is ideal for every patient and, indeed, during the average woman's reproductive lifetime of 30 or 40 years she is likely to need to use several techniques, for the requirements of the teenager are very different from those of the menopausal, multiparous grandmother. (Ramaswamy and Smith, 1976, p. 1)

> The contraceptive needs of a particular couple may undergo a series of changes during their reproductive lifetime. In the early days of their sexual relationship a couple may require maximum effectiveness . . . (IPPF, 1980, p. 53)

In the 'sexually active period before childbirth', when the need to prevent pregnancy is considered to be paramount, the pill or IUCD is thought to be appropriate. Less importance is attached to the avoidance of pregnancy when spacing births, so a method which is regarded as 'less reliable', such as the diaphragm, may be suggested. When childbearing is complete, sterilisation is considered to be a useful alternative to the pill or IUCD. It is possible that in discussions with patients about contraceptive use after completion of childbearing, doctors may stress the risks of the pill or IUCD which they did not emphasise earlier in the reproductive career.

In addition to these phases which hinge on the medical perception of the need to avoid pregnancy, there are three frequently described situations which occur at particular physiological developmental stages of the lifecycle that present special medical problems: the young girl in whom ovulation has not yet been established – contraindicating use of the pill; lactating women – for whom use of the combined pill may be contraindicated; and women aged 35 and over – for whom use of the pill becomes increasingly dangerous.

In each of these three situations, prevention of pregnancy is also considered essential – for medical, as well as social, reasons. The doctor is advised to balance the health risks of pregnancy with the reliability and health risks of the various methods. Use of relatively safe early abortion is not taken into this balance. Doctors are advised that in some cases the need to prevent pregnancy will outweigh the need to avoid possible side effects of a method.

Contraceptive needs are seen as changing within the reproductive lifetime which suggests a dynamic model of process. Instead, the identified stages are treated as discrete phenomena: women or couples who live through such life-histories move from one stage to another with no sense of past or future. Experience of methods is only considered to be useful information as a guide to motivation, though failure with a method is understood to create uncertainty about its reliability. Occasional examples suggest that, if asked, women would give ideas about past experience of methods and how it affects their current choices (Ramaswamy and Smith, 1976, p. 4; Guillebaud, 1975). This, then, is the strategy for contraceptive choice tied to the 'normal reproductive lifecycle'. The strategy is based on assumptions about the nature and social organisation of reproduction – that it should take place within marriage, that births should be spaced and limited, and that first childbirth should not be delayed too long since for women over 35 the risks of childbearing are increased for both her own health and the chance of abnormalities in the baby.

Conclusion

In spite of many appeals to the importance of the acceptability to the patient of the eventual method and the desirability that the patient should have all methods clearly explained and so be in a position to choose the method, it is clear that all the texts spend a great deal of time constructing ideal types of patients and matching them with appropriate methods. What is considered to be an appropriate method is based not only on physiological, medical factors but also on social and cultural factors. Indeed it is these latter aspects to which most of each text is devoted.

The historical development of the distinction between medical and social factors deserves further study. It is sufficient here to note that whereas the fight for contraception services in the 1950s centred on a more physiological interpretation of the proper concern of medicine, more recent debate reflects the growing concern of medicine as a whole with social aspects of medicine. 'Social factors' can be seen as being absorbed and interpreted by the medical profession in a similar way, for example, to biochemical or anatomical knowledge. Social attributes are seen as symptoms which can be incorporated in the search for a diagnosis.

What is at issue in the subject of contraceptive care is what constitutes the medical profession's body of knowledge about social factors. Doctors' perceptions of women's and men's contraceptive needs are based on assumptions about the social organisation of reproduction which support existing social and cultural norms. Medicine, in turn reinforces these norms, in its construction of 'patient choice'. Little attention is paid to the needs of women who might wish to have, or end up having, different reproductive histories. For example: women who do not wish to have children but do not want to be sterilised and who therefore face using contraceptive methods for 35 years or more, may experience dissatisfaction with these methods over a period of time; women who do not want to have children may find sterilisation difficult to obtain since it is assumed that all women want at least some children (Macintyre, 1976); women who want to postpone childbearing until the late 20s or early 30s and may not want to risk impairment of fertility with the pill or IUCD. The medical model of the contraceptive history does incorporate the idea of changing needs, but these variations are seen as resulting from the changing social *situation* of the individual rather than from changes in individual feelings and experiences.

Note

1. Midwives and nurses do play a role in family planning services, though this is usually one of supporting the doctor(s) rather than an independent role. This chapter concerns the literature written for the medical profession and does not include that written for the nursing and midwifery professions; the medical term 'patient' has therefore been used in preference to the nursing/midwifery term 'client'.

5 Sex and the Contraceptive Act
Scarlett Pollack

The standard of beautiful heterosexuality is the fulfilment of a man's desire and the assertion of his rights. It is within this context that contraceptives are researched, developed, distributed and used. Contraceptive methods are designed to fit in with, and protect this form of sexuality. Women are expected to accept it and conform by using contraceptives least likely to interfere with male-defined sex.

It is often argued that new technological developments in birth control have changed all this. Women's freedom from the burden and fear of unintended pregnancy is said to have been won by the widespread availability of reliable contraceptives. The joys of sex may therefore flourish without restraint. Women may now engage in sex on the same basis as men and, the argument continues, through contraceptive technology women have become the sexual equals of men. The sexual double standard is predicted to fade into history for its material basis, the possibility of pregnancy, is no longer reality in the lives of women and men. The technological separation of sex and reproduction, through the use of efficient contraceptives, achieves sexual liberation for women – or does it?

It is true, of course, that the range of contraceptives made widely available in recent years has offered greater alternatives for the prevention of pregnancy. This is a lever which has been used by women to negotiate for equality in heterosexual relationships. Women have increasingly come to view contraception as a right, for it provides a means necessary for choosing if, and when, to bear children. Greater choice over having children, and the possibility of having sex without becoming pregnant, have sometimes improved women's position within individual relationships. They have also made it more difficult for women to refuse men's sexual advances.

Use of the contraceptive pill and IUD (coil) by women has been beneficial for men. Freed from the responsibility and the practices involved in using the sheath or withdrawal, men have been able to concentrate more upon their enjoyment of sex. Yet the liberation of men from the use of contraceptives has had serious repercussions for women. First, women have been left with the responsibility for obtaining and using contraceptives. Second, men have easily absolved themselves from blame or responsibility, should the contraceptives fail to prevent pregnancy. Third, the most reliable methods of contraception have been associated with the highest health risks and side effects for women (Seaman and Seaman, 1978; Rakusen, 1981). Finally, women have continued to be the ones who face the consequences when things go wrong – when a pregnancy occurs and/or when health and comfort deteriorate.

Contraceptive technology does not provide the basis of sexual equality. What it does provide is a change. Potentially, contraceptives are as coercive as they are liberating. The gains and losses for women need to be analysed in view of the political relations into which new contraceptives are born.

Population control and family planning

The internationally funded and organised movement for population control has been concerned to distribute contraceptives as widely as possible. High priority is placed upon contraceptive methods which are reliable and cost effective, particularly in terms of service provision. The pill, IUD and more recently, the injectable Depo-Provera have been very popular in family planning organisations for these reasons – despite the known and suspected risks to the health and comfort of the women who use them (Vaughan, 1972; Seaman and Seaman, 1978; Rakusen, 1981).

Effectiveness of programmes is perceived as encouraging the use of reliable contraceptives and promoting small, stable family units. The health and welfare of women is a relatively minor side issue, except where ill health may interfere with women's ability to produce and raise children within the family structure. The question of women's rights or women's liberation is contrary to the objectives of population programmes. Both the IUD and Depo-Provera have been heralded for the 'advantage' that women have little control over them, once inserted or injected (Roberts, 1979, Rakusen, 1981). Whether in contraceptive decisions or plans to have children, the autonomy of women is in direct opposition to the stability of patriarchal family life.

Population control has two aspects: quantity and quality. Both the quantity of births and the quality of the population are at issue. Family planning programmes are directed specifically towards those women who are identified to be 'most at risk' of pregnancy. As all women who are engaging in sex with men, and are fertile, are at risk of pregnancy, the category 'at risk' is used very selectively. In practice it refers to those women identified by international policy makers, researchers and programme directors to be most in need of controlling the numbers of children they have. These women may be identified by the numbers of children they have, whether they are thought likely to exceed 'optimum family size', whether they have or are seen as likely to have children outside of marriage. They are also likely to be distinguished along racial, national and economic class lines (Gordon, 1977; Doyal, 1979). Political relations are central to the definitions, priorities and directions of population control programmes.

In Britain, the provision of contraceptive and abortion facilities has been firmly rooted in family planning. Concern to protect the patriarchal family structure has been pivotal to decisions about making birth control facilities available to women. Widespread provision of contraceptives for women was resisted on the grounds that freedom from fear of pregnancy would lead to promiscuity. This, in turn, would lead to the disruption and destruction of family life. Historically, the 'social grounds' in the fight for women's rights to contraceptives, abortion and sterilisation have had to be argued in terms of family stability in order to gain approval from both the medical profession and legislators. Arguments about overburdened and unwed mothers' needs to limit births gained a sympathetic ear, while debates about women's rights did not. Not surprisingly, proponents of birth control provision have usually stated their case in terms of the health and welfare of the family unit (Hindell and Simms, 1971; Greenwood and Young, 1976; Gordon, 1977; Lewis, 1980).

In the attempt to maintain the patriarchal family structure as the stable unit of society, fears of condoning women's 'promiscuity' have had to be weighed against the evidence of pregnancy and childbirth outside of marriage. The rising illegitimacy rates and illegal abortion figures of the 1960s were used to argue that the provision of birth control facilities was unavoidable if heterosexual family life were to be preserved. Both contraceptive and abortion facilities came about on this basis: the lesser of two evils (Greenwood and Young, 1976; Leathard, 1980). Sex education, too, found approval in the face of teenage pregnancy; even so, the emphasis has been much more upon the morals of family life and the mechanics of reproduction than it has upon practical sexual matters or contraception (Schofield, 1976; Farrell, 1978; Jackson, 1980).

Family planning is the form which population control takes. In the promotion of small families and the prevention of motherhood outside marriage, a reduction in the quantity of births is achieved, while the patriarchal family as the basic unit of social organisation is maintained. The international emphasis upon family planning supports family-based social orders, whilst diffusing the selective ways in which population control may be applied to various racial, national and economic groups.

In the field of family planning practice, Roberts (1981a) points out, there exists a male hegemony. It is men who control reproduction and women who are made to fit into male-defined categories. Male domination in the church and the state, the medical profession, research institutes and drug companies allows men, on an individual as well as an institutional level, to impose their perspective of women on women. Male-defined sexuality may be imposed upon women through this same system of male hegemony. Contraceptive research, distribution and use are designed to fit in with this order of sexuality, giving priority to male needs, wants and desires. The fact that it is women who become pregnant, give birth, experience contraceptive side effects, risk their health, undergo abortion, confront medical gatekeepers, and fall from social grace – while men are primarily concerned with their sexual pleasure – is made to appear trivial, if not invisible. The perspective of women which is imposed upon women is one which presents female contraceptive needs as female sexual needs, catering to the pleasure of her male partner.

Sex and power

It is not easy to talk about sex as an expression of power. Sexual intercourse is portrayed as an exchange of love or, at least, pleasure. It is said to be a free and spontaneous act, just doing what comes naturally. There are, of course, strict rules about where and when and why and how and with whom this spontaneity should take place.

Doing what comes naturally would seem to depend upon whether you are male or female. So do the social consequences of engaging in sexual relationships. Particularly outside of marriage, heterosexual partners are valued and treated very differently. It is an inverse relationship: sexual intercourse lowers a woman's social value and status at the same time as it heightens the status of her male partner. She becomes 'easy', 'loose' and 'cheap', while he is lauded for his virility. Sex makes her promiscuous while it proves him to be a man. Within the ideological disguise of a shared and loving sexual encounter there lurks a marked double standard of sexuality.

Male dominant practices define sex as something men do to women. Stevi Jackson (1982) points to the coercion which is built into sexual language and actions. Sex is something which women are said to react to. Men act and women react to what men do. This does not mean that women are not sexually active or active during sex. It does imply that women's actions are, or should be, geared primarily towards what men do, or don't do, and what men want. What turns men on, what excites men, what men feel, what men want women to do or be – is the focus of patriarchal sexual relations.

Whether or not love is involved, this is a political relationship. The differential power of men and women is clearly expressed in sexual relations. It is the privilege of men to be serviced sexually by women. This is not a reciprocal relationship, for sexual practices are oriented to men's pleasure while women's enjoyment is often ranked as an optional extra. While it may be within the capacity of individual men to grant or withhold women's enjoyment of sex, this is not taken to be a necessary part of what sex is.

The justification of sexual inequality hinges upon the belief that women like sex that way. A woman's sexuality is generally defined in terms of her partner's needs and desires: being able to sexually attract and excite him, give him affection and bear his children. From advertisements to pornography, from sexual innuendo to rape, images of sex depict women as enjoying and desiring the dominance of men. The conception of male virility is dependent upon female vulnerability and gratitude. Uppity women stand accused of creating an epidemic of male impotence (e.g. Frankl, 1975).

The sexual politics of contraception are revealed when women speak of their experiences, and are heard. Attempts by women to voice their experiences are more often met by denials, dismissals and justifications for patriarchal practices. The rhetoric of mutual loving relationships, in which sex is portrayed as an exchange between equals, hides more than it shows about sexual relations.

During my research on contraception I interviewed fifty women who were attending postgraduate courses at university and asked them about their experiences of sex and contraceptives. The women ranged in age from 23 to 38 years, and in duration of contraceptive use from six months to fifteen years. While there were many cultural differences amongst the women, most were white and from families of largely middle-class origin. Discussing their contraceptive decisions, the women related their experiences and feelings about sexual relationships. The myth of mutual sexuality was shattered by what women had to say about how sex was for them.

Most men, through ignorance or selfishness, appeared to expect women to enjoy what men enjoy about sex and to be satisfied with this. Women found it very difficult to confront this attitude, for men's feelings seemed to be easily hurt, or they became angry when women expressed what they felt. Rather than dealing with the inadequacy of male sexual definitions and practices for women, the 'problem' was most often seen to reside with the woman for making the man feel insecure or sexually inadequate. Male-oriented sex being the norm, women were aware of two things: first, that a partner who felt insulted or insecure might seek another woman who would accept his priorities; and second, that most men felt the same about sex.

For example, few of the women I talked with regularly experienced orgasms during love-making, although their partners almost invariably did. This is hardly surprising, for male orgasm is central to definitions and practices of what sex is; female orgasm is by-the-by, if at all. Women are not likely to experience orgasm when sex continues to be defined by men for men. Sexual intercourse is inadequate for women and hence, foreplay is essential. Yet, even the term 'foreplay' suggests a secondary-to-the-main-event activity, an optional extra:

> I tend to want a lot more time with it, a lot more exploratory work than a man normally tends to want or is often prepared to give.

Foreplay was not something which the majority of women felt they could expect from their partners. When it did play a part, it involved caressing and cuddling, but it was often neither clitoral nor oriented towards women's sexual satisfaction. Even during foreplay, women found that their pleasure was defined in terms of what their partner enjoyed. Foreplay usually turned out to mean before male orgasm; it included those activities which enhanced the man's pleasure. What was experienced as exciting to women was outside of the definition of sex, and women had difficulty even finding the language to talk about it:

> I only do (have an orgasm) in the course of conscious manipulations with the fingers or the tongue – in other words, while being masturbated by my partner rather than doing it myself. I'm not sure that's anything unusual, but it tends to be particularly conscious with me, rather than an automatic part of the way we make love.

Masturbation, as foreplay, carries the connotation of being a second-rate as well as secondary activity. That women felt compelled to describe their sexual arousal in these terms makes very clear that the definition of sex incorporates women only in relation to the sexuality of men. What happens after male orgasm, if anything, was even more difficult for women to find words to describe – afterplay?

The inequality of sex places a woman in a dependent and vulnerable position. Mutuality is not hers by right. Insofar as this depicts a loving relationship, the caring appears to flow primarily in one direction: from women to men. The marginality of what women actually experience and feel about this type of sexuality is more than a simple oversight on the part of men. Male eroticism is constructed upon the primacy of their wants and needs, and its justification rests upon the invisibility of how women actually feel about it. At the extreme this primacy may require physical force, but in everyday circumstances the ideology and practices of sex may be sufficient to affirm male dominant/female subordinate relations.

Beautiful oppression

Sex is, or should be, beautiful. Or should it? Standards of beauty have long been oppressive to women. The denial of reality in order to live up to men's expectations and desires is a constant theme of women's lives. Sexual attractiveness to men as a criterion of a woman's worth permeates every aspect of her life, and anything she may do. It is a criterion which tends to be positively correlated with gentleness, compassion, innocence and deference; and negatively associated with intelligence, aggression, ambition and achievement. What women do or say is judged in terms of whether men find it attractive and desirable.

Vulnerability and deference to men is central to patriarchal notions of womanliness and the beauty of the feminine stereotype. Aggressive, independent, or uncooperative women are by definition, unfeminine. What men find attractive is their relationship to women – the dominance they experience through their subordination of women.

Beautiful sex is the passionate embrace of masculinity and femininity. It is the embodiment of a romantic dream. Yet, for all its passion, sex is a neat and tidy package. Material reality is intrusive, complicating this patriarchal fantasy. Beautiful sex is not tinged with blood, discomfort, unintended pregnancy, or the need to discuss and use contraception. Reality is enough to put a man off.

A particularly clear example of this can be seen in male reactions to women menstruating. While the women I spoke with felt that the fact that they were menstruating ought to make little difference to their partner's sexual interest in them, many found that men recoiled at the idea. The sexual atmosphere was polluted by menstrual blood, men finding it sexually unattractive or even disgusting. Women often hoped that this attitude would pass as they got to know their partners better, but some were surprised to find it became worse:

> He never used to mind. But now if we're making love and he withdraws and it's sort of bloody or anything, he goes, 'Bleagh'. Or if I say I've got my period, he says, 'Oh, bloody hell' and gets a bit huffy about it. If I've got a tampon in and I have to go and take it out, I mean he doesn't like that at all.

While men were reluctant to discuss menstruation when sexual relations were 'new', the security of a long-term relationship seemed to allow them to fully express their feelings about menstruation. The reality of menstruation interfered with male perspectives of what beautiful and passionate sex is all about. Sophie Laws (in this volume) points out that pornographic images of women never include menstruation, for this is considered by men to be sexually off-putting.

Women found it easier to use contraceptives which helped to hide or minimise their menstrual blood. The pill, for example, was welcomed for its reduction of menstrual bleeding, while the diaphragm was valuable in holding menstrual blood, thus making it less visible to men. The coil, however, was a problem because of the increase in bleeding which women tended to experience when they used it. Patriarchal ideas conflicted with reality, and women were under pressure to hide that reality from men's eyes lest they be found to be sexually unappealing.

The contraceptive act

Beautiful heterosexuality is put into effect as the criterion against which women are judged by men. If a woman is interested in an individual man, in establishing a sexual relationship, then this is the standard with which she must be concerned. Whether she tries to conform to it, challenge or change it, she is faced with the expectation that she will look and act in a feminine manner – that is, in a way which is seen by men to be suitable for females. Only very carefully does she check out the possibility for change. For these are the rules, the behaviour he has come to expect.

'Interference' in sexual intercourse was highly problematic in the experience of the women I talked with. Both withdrawal and the sheath were seen as unacceptable methods to the extent that their male partners found sex to be less pleasurable when using them. The pill, being separate from the sexual event and not a hindrance to common patterns of sexual activities, was preferred – particularly by the men. Being able to separate the use of contraception from sexual intercourse, and the norms about sexual behaviour, was one of the three major considerations which women applied in taking decisions about birth control. In importance, it tended to override concern with side effects and health risks, while it was closely tied to considerations of reliability.

Ninety per cent of the women regarded using the contraceptive pill as possibly dangerous to their health. While ninety-four per cent had used it at some time, and sixty-four per cent were using it at the time I spoke with them, women's experiences with side effects reminded them of the risks they were taking. Frequently women thought about coming off the pill, or taking breaks from using it, but their male partners preferred them to use it. Men exerted pressure upon the women to go on the pill:

> He'd prefer me to go on the pill. It would be easier for him instead of stopping half-way.

to stay on it:

> I'm not happy about taking the pill. It's the simplest, but I thought the cap was quite safe. I've been thinking of taking a break but my husband said: 'Oh no, the smell of the cream was revolting' so I guess I won't go back even though I was quite satisfied really with the cap.

and to go back on it:

> He didn't like it one bit when I was having him use the sheath. He prefers me to damage my health with pills. He doesn't have to worry about that. He reckons it (the sheath) spoils all the fun.

Because those contraceptive methods which interfere least with sex are those which interfere most with women's health, the former is gained at the expense of the latter. The sexual perspective which gives priority to men's needs and desires is achieved at the expense of women's health and comfort.

Each of the alternatives to the pill was found to interfere with sexual norms and practices. The coil could be disruptive insofar as women experienced extended and heavier menstruation. The diaphragm and spermicides interfered with ideas about sexual spontaneity, requiring both planning and preparation. Use of withdrawal and the sheath needed discussion, care and confidence in the man's willingness and ability. The rhythm method involved an agreement about when sex is permissible, or the use of an alternative contraceptive method during 'unsafe' days. All of these contraceptive methods required planning, information, discussion and practical action – far from the romantic sweep of emotionality that beautiful sex is portrayed as.

Men tended to assume that their female partners would take the pill, or in some way be responsible for contraception. Women found it was left to them to raise the issue, to challenge their partner's assumptions or to insist upon alternative methods which were less convenient for men. Because women did not wish to lessen their partner's enjoyment of sex, they tended to deny their own needs and experiences, giving priority to those of men. It seemed easier, at least in the short run, to go along with the expectations of their partners and use the pill than to confront and challenge male dominant assumptions about sex and contraception.

The cap, or diaphragm, was seen by sixty-eight per cent of the women to interfere with sex. Many pointed to its 'premeditation' as the main disadvantage. In taking decisions about using the cap, acknowledging sex would or might occur was a factor to be weighed against the health risks of the pill and the coil:

> I don't like the premeditation bit about the cap but I think on the other hand, it's not interfering with any of your body processes, so that's an advantage. It's not upsetting the hormonal balance or inflicting heavy periods on yourself.

The fact that the cap is seen as less reliable than the pill or coil was, of course, another consideration. Women were uncertain, however, whether its ranking as less effective had to do with the method itself or with the temptation to use it without spermicides or, on occasion, not at all.

The premeditation of using the diaphragm tends to be seen very differently from the planning necessary when using the pill or coil. The proximity to individual sexual situations means that women are taking decisions each time they do, or think they will, have sex. This contradicts the patriarchal sexual scenario where women are believed to be the passive recipients of sex; here, innocent women are unexpectedly overcome by the passion to give in to a male sexual desire. Planning for sex would clearly imply women's knowledge and expectation, and undermine the female sexual dependence central to male dominant erotic fantasies. For men there is a direct contradiction between a woman's sexual appeal and her expectations and active plans for sex.

Acquiring sheaths involves a similar preparation for sex, yet it is viewed quite differently. Sheaths must be acquired in advance, made available at the time and place when sex happens, and their presence acknowledged by their use. But because obtaining sheaths is largely seen as a male activity, sexual ideology remains intact. Men in their assumed sexual knowledgeability are portrayed as the ones who expect, plan and execute sex.

However, men were not always found to be reliable in obtaining and using sheaths. In consequence, withdrawal would be used instead, increasing the woman's risk of becoming pregnant. It was this tension about the possibility of pregnancy which encouraged women to break the rules of sexual dependency by planning and taking contraceptive precautions themselves. This was easier when using a method which was separable from specific sexual encounters and in this respect, the pill and the coil were preferred to the diaphragm.

Contraceptive methods which are closely associated with sexual intercourse include withdrawal, the sheath, safe period, cap and spermicides – the majority of the available alternatives. To be used most effectively all of these contraceptives require information, discussion, planning and agreement between partners. Male dominant sexual ideology and practices conflict with this requirement. Emphasis upon romance and emotionality makes it difficult to have rational discussions and to reappraise the priorities of sex. This precludes the careful and flexible use of contraceptives. The concern of women for contraceptives which do not need to be used at the time of sexual intercourse is as much in pursuit of reliability as ease of use.

Control versus reponsibility

Nearly all of the women preferred to take contraceptive precautions themselves, rather than rely on their partners. This was connected with the greater reliability of female-centred methods, but over half of the women emphasised that being in control of whether the contraceptive was used was itself the most important consideration in assessing reliability. That is to say, whichever contraceptive method was used, its reliability depended upon whether women were influential over if and when and how it was used.

At the same time, women were concerned that this was allowing men to become increasingly irresponsible about contraception. Most men, they thought, were only too happy to leave women the responsibility for contraception. This was in part related to the method itself – specifically, the reliability of the pill and its non-interference with male-defined sexual intercourse. Yet, women were perturbed by a number of other factors which they identified in their partners' attitudes.

For one thing, the assumption that women using the pill were 'safe' from pregnancy, was at times used to imply that women were 'available'. That is, women felt under pressure that they should have sex whenever their partners wished. One way to challenge this attitude was to refuse to use the pill:

> I prefer not to let my partner assume he can have sex with me when he likes and it's going to be okay. I don't like to be abused, you know.

The presumption of women's sexual availability suggested a double irresponsibility on the part of the men: first, their irresponsible attitude towards taking contraceptive precautions led women to turn to female-centred methods; and second, the women's need for reliable contraceptives could be turned into a disadvantage by men.

A second factor which women detected in their partners was a willingness to disassociate themselves from the consequences of sex. If responsibility for contraception was assumed to belong to the woman, the man did not need to think about the possibility of pregnancy. Separating sex and reproduction, for men, meant that they were better able to concentrate upon their own sexual pleasure. Unlike women, they were freed of the responsibility for preventing unintended pregnancy:

> It's inclined to enable the man to totally forget he has any responsibilities whatsoever. It's no trouble for them. They don't have to know about it. They can just forget about it.

Female-centred contraceptives, with women taking responsibility for contraception and obtaining it, enabled men to distance themselves from the awareness of pregnancy and the responsibility for contraception.

In addition, women discovered that their partners, who had little of the responsibility for contraception, could easily claim no responsibility if things did not go according to plan. As the woman had organised and used the contraceptives, it was then said to be her fault and her problem should she become pregnant:

> Most men prefer the pill because it's easier and safe and it's no problem for them and they can blame me for it if anything goes wrong.

It must be noted, that even if the man takes the precautions, women tend to be the ones who are blamed, and whose responsibility it is for the pregnancy. As it is only men who are able to walk away from a pregnancy, the problem is ultimately the woman's, irrespective of contraceptive responsibility. Nevertheless, the tendency to leave contraception to women is convenient for men who wish to abdicate any responsibility for pregnancy.

Negotiating with men to achieve a more equal balance of responsibility was extremely difficult for women. The fact is that should mutual decisions, or even shared responsibility in contraceptive actions not work out, it is the woman who becomes pregnant. Still, many women tried to encourage their partners to be aware of, or share in, taking precautions to avoid pregnancy. The men were often less than willing:

> I decided to transfer responsibility to my partner for a while. But it's not really working out as I've had to buy them all (sheaths) so far. And he doesn't like it. If I'm not pregnant I think I might go back on the pill.

Combining men's irresponsibility about contraception with a greater reliability of methods such as the pill and the coil, convinced most of the women to use these methods in spite of the health risks involved.

Women looked to the future with great unease. The numerous years they envisaged needing contraception confronted them, while their experience of side effects increased over time. The health risks, too, became greater with length of use and with age, making future alternatives appear even fewer. Many of the women expressed a hope that in future, men would be able to use a male pill which would at least share out the risks taken between the two sexual partners. Once again, however, they were not sure their partners would be willing:

> He did say he wouldn't take a male pill as it may be physically harmful.

This woman was herself using the pill, despite concern about the effects on her health since 'there's no choice'. The refusal of men to endanger their own health by using methods which they find acceptable for their women partners to use, clearly revealed their concern to protect the privileges of men.

Similarly, the question of sterilisation brought out men's attitudes towards the primacy of their sexual feelings over the health risks women were taking. Although vasectomy is a much less hazardous operation than female sterilisation, many of the women's partners found the idea objectionable, with the consequence that either women would go on taking contraceptive risks or undergo sterilisation themselves. As one woman explained:

> My husband's against vasectomy adamantly. He's just so squeamish. He can't stand the thought of anyone coming near him with a scalpel, particularly near his balls, so he just won't even contemplate that.

Years of taking risks with methods of contraception led many women to the hope, if not the expectation, that their partners would be willing to take responsibility by accepting vasectomy in the future. Concern about male feelings of virility, and psychological insecurity, however, left women sceptical of their chances of active male support over contraceptive issues when the time came.

Summary

The inequality of sexuality provides the basis for contraceptive activities. New technologies are developed from a patriarchal perspective, emphasising the sexual enjoyment of men and underestimating the costs to women. Male sexual pleasure is the most significant factor taken into account in the methods which become available, and in the ways in which contraceptives are used.

Sexual practices which conform to male standards, while denying women's experience of sex, are justified by the assumption that women are satisfied with male dominant sex. The dominance of men itself is believed to satisfy women sexually. This can only be maintained, however, by rendering invisible women's feelings, experiences and objections. Contraceptive practices are very similar. Undermining women's experiences of contraceptives, and male attitudes towards contraception, result in the inevitable appearance of contraceptive inequalities.

The socially subordinate position of women places our concerns about contraception amidst a body of ideas and practices which affirm men's privilege to be serviced sexually by women. The sexual desires of men are given priority over their consequences for women, and over the desires of women. Contraceptive side effects and health risks to women are presented as of relatively minor significance. Taken-for-granted notions about contraception, like sex, are much more comfortable for men to live with than for women. Contraception, for women, is self-defence. To be most effective it must involve a reassessment of sexual priorities, a redefinition of the criteria of contraception, and the assertion of women's experiences and concerns.

6 Legal Abortion in Great Britain

Madeleine Simms

Abortion is the central feminist issue of our time, as birth control was for the previous generation, and suffrage for the generation before that. This chapter traces the social and political history of the Abortion Act from the 1930s onwards. It discusses the changes the Act brought about, the problems it revealed, and the solutions that were devised to try to overcome them. The subsequent development of the abortion services is outlined together with details of the political campaign against legal abortion led by militant religious pressure groups. The chapter concludes by looking forward to the time when abortion ceases to be a political issue.

The Abortion Act was passed in October 1967 and came into effect in April 1968. This marked the culmination of a campaign for abortion law reform which had lasted more than 30 years (Hindell and Simms, 1971).

The early years of the campaign

The Abortion Law Reform Association was founded in 1936 by a group of women, most of whom had been involved in other progressive causes of the period. Some had campaigned for votes for women 25 years earlier, some had been active in the birth control cause, some had been involved in the work of the Labour Party, and several were active Freethinkers. They were aware that there had been a striking improvement in public health since the First World War. In his Annual Report for 1933 the Chief Medical Officer of the Ministry of Health had observed that the mortality from tuberculosis had been halved during the last 20 years, a reduction comparable with the decline in infant mortality (HMSO, 1934). This provided a striking contrast with maternal mortality:

> For twenty years that rate has remained static at or about 4 deaths per 1,000 births. (HMSO, 1934, p. 259)

He said that one reason for this was:

> A substantial increase in abortion, and in the habit of abortion . . . which is now materially affecting maternal mortality. (HMSO, 1934, p. 261)

In 1933, 463 women died as a direct result of abortion. Another 97 women died for reasons 'associated with abortion'. These were the official figures. The Chief Medical Officer recognised that these figures were incomplete and that additional deaths took place from abortion that were ascribed to other more respectable causes. The social stigma then attached to the subject ensured its systematic under-reporting.

Whereas birth control had always been legal, under The Offences Against the Person Act, 1861, abortion was illegal in England and Wales. However, a small but increasing number of abortions were performed in public hospitals where the woman's life was in danger. At the same time, middle class women bought abortions privately from expensive doctors, while working class women bought them more cheaply and more dangerously from illegal abortionists who, although unqualified, were often quite experienced. By contrast to England and Wales, in Scotland it had long been possible for a doctor to carry out an abortion if it was necessary in his clinical judgement. A doctor could not be charged with illegal abortion unless a specific complaint had been brought against him and there was evidence that he had not acted in good faith. In practice, however, abortions were probably carried out on much the same grounds as in England, though there were variations within Scotland according to local religious tradition.

Nobody knew how many illegal abortions took place each year. Estimates varied from about 50,000 a year (Birkett Committee, 1939) to 250,000 a year (Chesser, 1949). Meanwhile, without benefit of modern contraception, birth rates fell relentlessly. In 1933, the birth rate in England and Wales fell to 14 per 1,000, the lowest figure ever recorded until that time. This too caused public and professional anxiety. The medical profession and the government set up committees to investigate the abortion problem.

The British Medical Association published its *Report on the Medical Aspects of Abortion* in 1936. It recommended that abortion should be legal where it was necessary to preserve the physical or mental health of the mother, where sexual assault had taken place or where the baby would be likely to be born abnormal. It aroused much controversy by also suggesting that 'the community as a whole', and not just the medical profession, ought to consider whether abortion should be legalised 'for social and economic reasons' (BMA, 1936).

In 1937, the government appointed a committee under Mr Norman Birkett, KC, later a High Court judge, to inquire into abortion. The committee was dominated by a group of eminent and conservative doctors and its conclusions were correspondingly cautious (Birkett Committee, 1939). It confined itself to recommending that abortion should be legalised where this was necessary to preserve the life or health of the mother. However, one member of the Birkett Committee, Dorothy Thurtle, a Labour Party politician, went further. She recognised, even then, that early, medically induced abortion was at least as safe as childbirth itself. Recent experience in the Soviet Union had demonstrated this. She therefore recommended that abortion also be made legal in cases of sexual assault, where the baby might be born abnormal, and where the women had already had four pregnancies.

While this committee was sitting, a notable trial took place which was to have a great impact on public opinion. A 14 year old girl had been assaulted and raped by two soldiers. A courageous gynaecologist, Mr Aleck Bourne, agreed to carry out an abortion, and informed the police of his action as he did not wish to be accused of acting illegally. He was arrested amid much publicity. After a long trial he was acquitted on the grounds that the original 1861 Act referred to instances when abortion was 'unlawful' and therefore it followed that it must sometimes also be lawful. An obvious instance was when the woman's life was at stake. However, it was not possible to distinguish between danger to life and danger to health. Thus, the judge concluded, abortion must be lawful if the pregnancy would otherwise severely damage a woman's physical or mental health. The Bourne judgement greatly liberalised English abortion law, even though it was only a single case and did not go to the Appeal Court. There still remained some doubts that a higher court might reverse this judgement, though as time went by and the Bourne judgement was reinforced by further legal cases, these fears lessened.

Parliamentary activity begins

During the Second World War all abortion law reform activities ceased. In 1951, however, the abortion issue was sharply revived when the Pope, in a speech delivered to Italian midwives, repeated the Church's traditional objection to birth control, adding that abortion was never justified, not even to save the life of the mother. This announcement was very badly received, even by leading members of the Church of England, in the more radical post-war atmosphere that prevailed in Britain. The next year, 1952, Mr Joseph Reeves, a Labour MP, introduced the first of what were to be six parliamentary bills which attempted to reform the antiquated abortion laws. All abortion bills in Britain have been introduced into Parliament by individual Members of Parliament and not by governments, which do not wish to get actively involved in such controversial matters. Since little parliamentary time is available for such private legislation, Members of Parliament enter a ballot once a year and only those who are fortunate enough to come out near the top of the list (usually the first eight names) can hope to obtain enough parliamentary time not only to introduce a measure in the House of Commons, but also to guide it through all the necessary stages until it becomes law. Mr Reeve's bill failed, and was succeeded in 1961 by another attempt, by Mr Kenneth Robinson, MP, who was to become Labour Minister of Health a few years later. Roman Catholic MPs of all parties combined to defeat this measure, but now against a rising tide of public opinion which the Abortion Law Reform Association was helping to organise outside Parliament by publicity and political lobbying.

It was at this point that the thalidomide tragedy occurred. Pregnant women had taken drugs prescribed by their doctors to combat nausea in pregnancy, and now they learned that these drugs sometimes caused severe deformities in babies. When some pregnant women who had taken this drug requested legal abortions they were informed that though the prescription they had been given was legal, the proposed abortion was illegal. This argument immediately swept the abortion issue into the arena of public health and it ceased to be associated solely with criminal and surreptitious activities. It also swept a new and energetic generation into the Abortion Law Reform Association, determined to bring about a more liberal and humane law. On 25 July 1962, a London national newspaper, the *Daily Mail*, published a startling public opinion poll showing that 73 per cent of the public was in favour of abortion where a child might be born deformed. The thalidomide tragedy educated a new generation into the realities of the abortion situation. Many new and useful drugs were coming onto the market that might nonetheless be found subsequently to produce unexpected and dreadful side effects. Abortion needed to be made widely available at least on health grounds to take account of this development. Many couples in the childbearing groups felt concerned about this. Two further parliamentary bills were introduced into the House of Commons, one by a Labour MP, Mrs Renée Short, and another by a Conservative MP, Mr Simon Wingfield Digby. Again they were defeated by the Catholic MPs of all parties who spoke so long in the debate that allotted parliamentary time ran out. But these parliamentary tactics were now openly criticised by people in all political parties.

When Lord Silkin introduced the first abortion bill into the House of Lords in 1965 he was surprised at the good progress it made in the now altered state of public opinion. A general election intervened which brought his bill to an end, but he successfully re-introduced it in the new session of Parliament. In 1966, however, Mr David Steel, a young Scottish Liberal MP, who in later years was to become leader of the Liberal Party, drew third place in the Private Members' ballot and agreed to introduce a bill in the House of Commons to liberalise the abortion law, thus causing Lord Silkin to withdraw his own bill in the House of Lords in favour of Mr Steel's. The bill was opposed by the more right wing Conservative MPs and by Roman Catholic MPs of all parties, as was now the established pattern of opposition to abortion law reform. At the same time the bill was supported by a large number of non-Catholic Labour MPs, by a small number of the more progressive Conservative MPs, as well as by most of the small number of Liberal MPs. The struggle to bring the bill to a successful conclusion was a long and arduous one. The by now very experienced Lord Silkin guided Mr Steel's bill through its various stages in the House of Lords. So bitter was the opposition that the bill nearly ran out of time but the Labour Government, which was on the whole sympathetic to abortion law reform, agreed to allow some additional government time to permit the debate to finish and the necessary votes to be taken. The bill finally passed into law on 27 October 1967 and came into operation on 27 April 1968.

It is always difficult to pinpoint why a particular piece of reforming legislation comes about in one decade rather than another. The Second World War had unleashed radical forces in British domestic politics. The urge towards greater social equality and justice for all sections of society was partly embodied in the programme of the first post-war Labour government with its emphasis on public ownership, social security and the establishment of the National Health Service, legal aid and the children's services. The social legislation of the 1960s was probably the final manifestation of the aspirations and optimism of this post-war era. This was also, of course, an era of unprecedented prosperity for this country. Despite a series of economic crises, there was full employment, a rapidly rising standard of living, and confidence in the future – a strikingly different world from that of the 1980s. Social confidence allows compassion, generosity and innovation to flourish. It creates an ambience which is sympathetic to social reform and experiment.

Another feature of the 1960s which is not often remarked upon is that it contained the first substantial generation of women graduates. Many of these educated women were now sitting at home with young children, wondering what to do with their lives. John Bowlby and fellow child psychiatrists seemed to be warning women against becoming working mothers (Bowlby, 1952). A considerable number of these young, housebound, graduate married women, many with young children, formed the core of the revitalised Abortion Law Reform Association, and many other similar reforming groups, which became such formidable campaigning organisations in the 1960s. These women were feminists, but not by present day standards very liberated. Their spare time activities were subsidised by their husbands' earnings, not their own. The Women's Movement – the third wave of modern feminism – was in its early days and the abortion law reform movement owed nothing to it as yet.

With the advent of the contraceptive pill, birth control was almost universally practised by married couples, and increasingly by the unmarried also. The Brook Advisory Centres were established during this period to cater for the contraceptive needs of young women in their late teens and early twenties.

Religious practice had become a minority preoccupation and the Roman Catholic Church was in growing disarray over its social morality. Catholics were now openly using birth control by methods forbidden by their Church, and this was causing heated public debate.

The reform of the abortion laws was increasingly seen as a logical extension of other methods of fertility control. National Opinion Polls carried out a national abortion survey in 1965 which showed that 75 per cent of Anglicans, 68 per cent of Nonconformists, 65 per cent of Presbyterians, and even 60 per cent of Roman Catholics all favoured a measure of abortion law reform. Doctors' opinions too were changing rapidly. The majority of general practitioners were known to favour a liberal abortion law, though this grass roots view had not yet penetrated the rarified atmosphere of the Royal Colleges. But then it was the family doctors, not the specialists, who were in the front line and had to face the patients who were desperate for terminations.

Finally, and perhaps most important of all, was the composition of the Labour back benches after the 1966 General Election. This brought 363 Labour MPs into the House of Commons, the highest number since 1945, of whom more than half were university graduates and nearly 100 were teachers, dons, writers or journalists. Moreover, nearly 100 were in their twenties or thirties. They wanted to see action. Abortion was one of a number of obvious social reforms, where the state of the law was absurdly antiquated and widely ignored. Additionally, it was also an inexpensive reform. Indeed, it was one that, properly considered, would actually save public money in the long run by reducing the numbers of septic abortions requiring hospital treatment. Here, surely, was a reform whose time had come, and the Labour intake of the mid 1960s was composed of a high proportion of liberal minded intellectuals who would be eager to take advantage of this fact.

The 1967 Abortion Act

How did the Abortion Act change the situation? It confirmed that abortion was legal where it was necessary to preserve the physical or mental health of the mother. This ground had already been established by the 1938 Bourne judgement, but now it was strengthened by being turned into statute law. Legal abortion was also extended to avoid the birth of a seriously handicapped child. There were two important innovations. In the first place, a medico-social clause was introduced. The effect of the pregnancy on the 'existing children of the family' could be taken into account by doctors, as could the woman's social environment (Abortion Act 1967). In the early years of the abortion law reform campaign, the argument had centred mainly on health issues. But social issues became increasingly important in the later stages of the debate. The extreme difficulty in distinguishing medical from social grounds in the context of both birth control and abortion became recognised, and found expression in this wording of the Act. The second innovation came about as a result of intervention by the Lord Chief Justice who wanted a clear criterion for judges when trying abortion cases in the courts. Abortion was held to be legal if it was safer for the woman than continuing with the pregnancy (House of Lords Debates, 1967). Opponents of legal abortion allowed this principle to be incorporated into the Act because they genuinely believed abortion to be an extremely dangerous operation. As early abortion carried out by qualified doctors in medical settings became increasingly safer than childbirth, the importance of this aspect of the Abortion Act grew.

The Abortion Act also contained three constraints which were new to the abortion situation in Britain. All abortions had to be notified to the Chief Medical Officer at the Department of Health. Not one, but now two doctors had to agree to the abortion and sign the necessary documents. The abortion had to be carried out in a National Health Service hospital or a private clinic 'approved' by the Minister. This meant that the private clinics had to be licensed and inspected by government officials.

These regulations were not welcomed by all abortion law reformers for they hedged the abortion operation with rules that did not apply to other much more dangerous surgical procedures. The regulations were restrictive in intention and thus strongly supported by the Act's opponents who argued that this degree of medical and civil service supervision would reduce the likelihood of abortion 'abuses' occurring. The reformers who saw quite clearly the intentions that lay behind these regulations, regarded them as part of a necessary price to be paid for obtaining some reform of the law. It was a compromise, but a worthwhile one, given the benefits to women that the Abortion Act brought in its wake.

The shape of the abortion services

In 1969, the first calendar year after the Abortion Act came into effect, some 50,000 legal abortions were notified in England and Wales for British women. This number doubled within the next two years and remained, with fluctuations, at between 100,000 and 130,000 for the next twelve years (Table 1). In Scotland, about 7,500 abortions were carried out each year from 1972 (SHHD, 1981, p. 309) and about 1,000 women travelled annually from Scotland to England for

Table 1 Abortions in England and Wales on British Residents

Year	*Number of abortions for women of all ages*
1971	94,600
1972	108,600
1973	110,400
1974	109,600
1975	106,200
1976	101,900
1977	102,700
1978	111,900
1979	120,600
1980	128,900
1981	128,600
1982	128,600

Source: 1984: *OPCS Population Trends*, no. 36, p. 62.

abortion, mostly from the Catholic Glasgow area where abortions were difficult to obtain (OPCS, 1981, p. 52). In addition, increasing numbers of foreign women came to London from other countries in Europe to obtain medically performed abortions which were still illegal in their own countries. This reached a peak of 56,500 in 1973 when 35,300 French and 11,300 West German women came to England for abortions (Tietz, 1983, p. 36). As French and German abortion laws were reformed these numbers dropped sharply and Italian and Spanish women took the place of the French and the Germans. The Abortion Act did not apply to Northern Ireland where abortion remained illegal except on narrow medical indications. So each year more women from Northern Ireland (and from the Irish Republic) came to England for abortion. Many stayed with English friends and relations and were entered in the English abortion statistics. Between 1972 and 1974, one third of all abortions performed in England and Wales were carried out on women from overseas, but this proportion declined in the late 1970s.

Foreign women had to obtain their abortions in the private sector of medicine and so increasingly did British women. In 1969, more than 60 per cent of British women in England and Wales who had abortions obtained them in the National Health Service. But this proportion fell steadily. The National Health Service continued to carry out between 50–58,000 abortions each year from 1971 to 1978, while the increase in demand was catered for in the private sector (Lewis, 1980, p. 296). In 1980, 60,000 (46 per cent) British women had a National Health

Service abortion; while 70,000 had a private abortion in one of the 60 private nursing homes approved for abortion, as did more than 30,000 foreign women (OPCS, 1981, p. 1). By contrast, within Scotland nearly all abortions were carried out in the National Health Service, but about 15 per cent of all Scottish abortion patients annually travel to England to obtain abortions, mostly in the private sector (OPCS, 1981, p. 52). Overall, however, the abortion rate for Scottish women is somewhat lower than for women in England and Wales.

Since the early years following the Act, abortion services have been unevenly distributed around the country. In 1969 there were six NHS abortions in the city of Newcastle for every 100 live births, whereas in Birmingham there were only two per 100. Ten years later there were 12 NHS abortions per 100 live births in Newcastle, but still only one third of this rate in Birmingham. This was because many doctors in Birmingham were opposed to the Abortion Act and refused to perform abortions, whereas doctors in Newcastle had been sympathetic and had a long tradition of carrying out abortions on health and medico-social grounds, even before the Abortion Act was passed. Similar contrasts prevailed in Scotland. Legal abortion on medico-social grounds had been carried out for very many years in the Aberdeen area under the famous gynaecologist, Sir Dugald Baird. In Glasgow, with its large Roman Catholic population, few abortions were carried out and women had to travel outside the city for their abortions, particularly to Edinburgh where the influx of Glasgow abortion patients created problems for local medical services (*Edinburgh Sunday Standard*, 1981). These disparities arose because legal abortion was not available at the request of the woman, but only on the recommendation of the doctors.

Soon after the Abortion Act was passed it became apparent that even though abortion was now legal in many circumstances, this did not make it much easier for women to obtain legal and safe abortions in those parts of the country where doctors disapproved of abortion on moral or religious grounds, or had no extra facilities with which to carry out abortions even if they were willing in principle to do so. This situation persuaded several members of the Abortion Law Reform Association to come together to set up independent non-profit referral agencies and later clinics of their own. The first of these Pregnancy Advisory Services was established in Birmingham, where the professor of gynaecology at the University hospital and many of his staff were opposed to abortion law reform and where women had great problems about obtaining abortions. In later years a similar service was established in London. By the mid 1970s between 30,000 and 40,000 abortions were being carried out each year under the auspices of the British Pregnancy Advisory Service and the Pregnancy Advisory Service, London. Nearly all of these were carried out on British women (BPAS,

1978). Thus, more than half of all British women who obtained legal abortions in the private sector of medicine, obtained their operations through the abortion charities. This is a development of great interest in the field of social medicine because the abortion charities are ultimately controlled by consumers, not by doctors.

In Britain, the 1960s and 1970s were a period of great development in the consumer movement in several fields. Consumers wished to increase their bargaining power in relation to producers who often supplied poor quality, expensive or dangerous goods. Now this movement had spread into the medical field and, despite considerable opposition and interference by hostile doctors and hostile governments, the pregnancy advisory services thrived because they answered an urgent need on the part of patients who could not be accommodated in the National Health Service and could not afford expensive fees in the commercial private sector of medicine. Moreover, because of their emphasis on abortion counselling and the needs of women, the abortion charities developed a good reputation among the younger generation and as their reputation increased, the number of their clients grew. The abortion charities were an important source of innovation not only in the field of abortion counselling but also in the development of day-care abortion services, 'morning-after' contraception and other forms of client-centred care. Now some health authorities are beginning to contract out their abortion clients to these charities, which carry out the operations free of charge to the client, expenses being met by the health authority.

Results of reform

In the decade before the passing of the Abortion Act, between 50 and 60 women died annually in England as a result of abortion; now less than 10 per cent of this number die. In 1979 the government published a table (BPAS, 1979) for a parliamentary committee, showing that whereas other maternal deaths had fallen by about half, maternal deaths due to abortion had fallen by nearly 90 per cent (Table 2). Discharges from hospitals following a diagnosis of septic abortion fell by more than 3,000 in 1968 to 500 in the mid 1970s (BPAS, 1978). During this period abortion offences known to the police fell from 247 to 11 (BPAS, 1978) and the numbers of persons found guilty of procuring illegal abortion fell from 60 to 2 (BPAS, 1978).

Abortion mortality is greatly affected by length of gestation. In England and Wales in 1978, 83 per cent of abortions were carried out in the first trimester of pregnancy, another 13 per cent between 13 and 16 weeks, and 4 per cent at 17 weeks or more (Tietz, 1983). About 1.5 per cent of all abortions are carried out at 20 weeks or later. A handful of these, 281 in 1979, were carried out at 24 weeks or over (House of Commons Debates, 1980). These very late abortions have been the

Table 2 Maternal Deaths 1968–1978 England Only

Year		*1968*	*1969*	*1970*	*1971*	*1972*	*1973*	*1974*	*1975*	*1976*	*1977*	*1978*
Maternal deaths due to abortion (all types)	(a)	48	34	29	26	23	10	9	5	6	6	5
Other maternal deaths	(b)	143	113	108	103	85	66	64	62	68	66	65
Total maternal deaths	(a + b)	191	147	137	129	108	76	73	67	74	72	70
Per cent of all maternal deaths due to abortion (all types)		25	23	21	20	21	13	12	7	8	8	7

Source: BPAS, 1979.

focus of much political controversy over the years. Those who tend to have later, and therefore more dangerous, abortions include women born abroad, the very young, and women from the lowest social class. Even women normally resident in England, but who were born in the West Indies, India and Pakistan are ten times more likely to die from abortions than are women actually born in Great Britain (DHSS, 1979b). These are women who may have more difficulty in finding out where to obtain a legal abortion, and securing the necessary two medical signatures required by law.

Only some 2 to 3 per cent of all abortions are undertaken to prevent the birth of a seriously handicapped baby. In 1978, about 1,500 abortions were carried out on these grounds alone, and another 1,000 abortions on these grounds combined with others (OPCS Monitors, 1979). The fact, however, that abortion is now legal where serious abnormality is expected, has encouraged research into methods of detecting such conditions and it is anticipated that these grounds for legal abortion may assume greater importance in the future as methods of prediction continue to improve.

A government committee investigates

Successive governments found themselves harassed by the abortion conflict. In 1971, the then Conservative government decided to set up a Committee of Enquiry into the Abortion Act to see whether there were any serious problems about its working that needed correcting. The government appointed as chairman of the committee the only woman High Court judge, the Honourable Mrs Justice Elizabeth Lane. Doctors, psychiatrists, lawyers, social workers, health administrators and teachers sat on the committee and spent three years investigating all aspects of the abortion services. Despite the fact that this committee had been established in response to complaints about legalised abortion and on the initiative of opponents of reform, the committee came to very positive conclusions about the effects of the Abortion Act:

> By facilitating a greatly increased number of abortions the Act has relieved a vast amount of individual suffering . . . We are unanimous in supporting the Act and its provisions. We have no doubt that the gains facilitated by the Act have much outweighed any disadvantages for which it has been criticised. (Lane Committee, 1974, p. 184)

The Lane Committee did not recommend any alterations to the grounds of the Abortion Act, but did recommend that there should be an upper time limit of 24 weeks' gestation for legal abortion and made a large number of administrative suggestions of which the most important was that there be an extension of day-patient surgery. The research commissioned by the government's Lane Committee and published as Volume III of the Lane Report had established that 87 per cent of women sought abortion in the first two months of pregnancy. The delays that took place were attributable to doctors and the health system, not patients. Thus the committee concluded:

> The speed of the (day-care) procedure should enable waiting lists to be reduced and thus make it possible to operate earlier in pregnancy when the risks of mortality and morbidity are lower. (Lane Committee, 1974, p. 147)

The conclusions of the Lane Committee were carefully moderate. The committee did not recommend that the abortion decision be placed in the hands of the woman herself instead of her doctor, as feminists hoped. But neither did the committee recommend any serious restrictions. This came as a great blow to opponents of the Abortion Act who were determined to obtain by directly political means what they had failed to achieve by recommendation of an impartial survey.

The political controversy over the Abortion Act

Attacks on the Abortion Act started almost as soon as it was passed. Between 1969 and 1982 there were eight attempts by opponents of reform to restrict the Abortion Act. Five of these were made by Conservative MPs, one by a Labour MP representing a heavily Catholic constituency, another by a Roman Catholic Liberal MP and another by a member of the House of Lords. All these attempts failed, though sometimes by very narrow majorities. Supporters of the Abortion Act used all possible parliamentary devices to prevent any proposed restrictions from passing into law. Just as Catholic MPs had in the past prevented abortion law reform coming about by talking so long that votes could not be taken, so now their opponents sometimes used the same tactics to save the Abortion Act from being destroyed.

Parliamentary attempts to restrict the Abortion Act have taken several forms. Some MPs have tried to impose legal time limits at 20, 22 or 24 weeks' gestation. Others have tried to insist that only senior doctors or specialists could sign the abortion certificates, a step that would have the effect of causing long delays so that many women would have been denied abortions. Attempts have been made to curb the abortion charities and to destroy the connection between their referral agencies and their clinics. Some MPs have sought to strengthen those sections of the Abortion Act that enable medical and nursing staff with conscientious objections to abortion to refuse to take part in the abortion services. A few have even tried to alter the very grounds for legal abortion, removing the social grounds for abortion, or changing the provision relating to abortion being legal when the more dangerous alternative is to continue with the pregnancy.

The Abortion Law Reform Association recognised that with each year of its existence, the abortion law would be strengthened and more likely to survive. Abortion law reformers argued that the fall in abortion deaths, the fall in the number of septic abortions reaching hospitals, and the fall in the number of criminal abortion cases known to the police, have resulted directly from the passing of the 1967 Abortion Act. But those opposed to reform usually ascribed these benefits to other causes such as advances in medicine or reduced police vigilance.

The medical profession as a whole was impressed by the health benefits it believed to have resulted from the Abortion Act. Whereas official representatives of the medical profession had opposed the passing of the 1967 Abortion Act, ten years later the medical profession was to fight actively to preserve this legislation. The Abortion Act has gradually converted not only the medical profession, but also a number of other social work and ancillary professions. These came together in 1976 to form the Co-ordinating Committee in Defence of the 1967 Abortion Act (Co-ord, 1981). By 1980, more than 50 organisations were members of this Committee, including associations from all political parties and a national religious organisation called Christians for Free Choice.

At the same time, powerful religious groups had developed in opposition to the Abortion Act. These aimed to weaken, restrict or, if possible, destroy it. Two of these groups, the Society for the Protection of the Unborn Child (*SPUC*) and *Life* developed large national organisations and received much support from the Roman Catholic Church and one wing of the Church of England. They held large demonstrations against the Abortion Act and organised intense parliamentary lobbying. *Life* has also established associated counselling and welfare agencies that seek to dissuade women from having abortions and offer them social support and housing if they agree to continue with the pregnancy.

Meanwhile, the Women's Movement gained strength in Britain throughout the 1970s and in response to what it saw as the anti-feminist activities of these groups, it established its own National Abortion Campaign which developed close links with the trade union movement and the women's sections of the Labour Party. This introduced a new and important element into the political struggle to preserve legal abortion. Once the trade unions and Labour women were involved it became increasingly difficult for even the Roman Catholic Labour MPs to actively support any restriction of the Abortion Act. Moreover, the National Abortion Campaign had groups throughout the country and was less London-centred than the Abortion Law Reform

Association. It was therefore able to exert its pressure more widely, particularly in the larger provincial cities.

Discussion

What picture emerges after 17 years of legal abortion in Britain? Early and safe abortion appears to be much more widely available to working class women than in the past (Dunnell, 1979) though, allowing for the 20 per cent increase in the population during the past half century, there is no convincing evidence that the total numbers of abortions have increased disproportionately, nor that the ratio of induced abortions to live births has greatly altered (Simms, 1981). Since most abortions carried out before the Abortion Act were illegal, it will never be known with any certainty what the actual numbers were. All one can be certain of is that illegal abortion was considered a major social and medical problem in the past and is now no longer considered so. In 1935 Parish, a London gynaecologist, published a paper on 1,000 abortion cases treated in his hospital (Parish, 1935). He had no doubt that illegal abortion was increasing rapidly. In 1949, Simpson observed that the 500 abortion deaths occurring each year were not a true reflection of the actual incidence of abortion, which he believed to be very high.

> The principle dangers of abortion will remain unchanged so long as it is unlawful to induce it for mere social and economic reasons. (Simpson, 1949, pp. 47–9)

Another London gynaecologist, Davis, estimated in 1950 that 90 per cent of all abortions reaching hospital were illegally induced, often by the woman herself, by a variety of dangerous methods which he discussed in detail (Davis, 1950, pp. 123–30). At the same time, of course, many illegal abortions were quite successfully induced and required no subsequent admission to hospital.

There have, of course, been many other developments during the past half-century that have had an important bearing on the abortion situation, notably improvements in public education and in the free birth control services made available under the National Health Service (contraceptives became available without charge in 1974). These must have reduced the actual need for abortion on the part of many women. At the same time, there have been improvements in working opportunities for women which may have had the effect of greatly raising expectations about effective fertility control, and thus actually increasing the demand for abortion services where birth control has failed. What is certain, however, is that there has been a great increase in the use of birth control during recent years (Cartwright, 1978) and a sharp fall in abortion deaths, septic abortions, and illegal abortions known to the police.

Nonetheless, there is still an unmet need for abortion, though it is not possible to say how large this is. The Lane Committee came to the conclusion that the average acceptance rate in the National Health Service was 70 per cent. It thought that probably about one third of those women at first refused abortion, obtained abortion elsewhere. But, of course, some, perhaps many, abortion seekers never reach a National Health Service hospital. In the National Health Service, the patient first has to consult her family doctor about her abortion and then she is referred to the specialist at the local hospital if the GP thinks there is a case for abortion under the terms of the Abortion Act. This procedure allows the family doctor a great deal of discretion in how the Abortion Act is interpreted, according to his or her own religious or moral beliefs. These considerations also come into play when the woman has reached the hospital specialists (Allen, 1981; Ashton, 1980). Hence the wide regional variation in NHS abortion that has been such a feature of the abortion scene in Britain since the Act was passed. Even now it is three times more difficult for women in some hospital regions to obtain NHS abortions than in others. In some districts, virtually no NHS abortion is available at all and women who require an abortion have to buy it privately or else continue with an unwanted pregnancy.

A decade after the recommendations of the Lane Committee, the National Health Service has still not been able to adapt to providing a fast, efficient national abortion service. A committee of the Royal College of Obstetricians and Gynaecologists reported in 1984:

> Objective measures of delay suggest that deficiencies in the organisation of the abortion service, especially in the NHS, make a substantial contribution to avoidable delay in second trimester abortion . . . (Alberman and Dennis, 1984, p. 105)

The authors pointed out that a substantial proportion of women who had to undergo late abortions, had consulted a doctor very early in pregnancy but then became caught up in a slow, bureaucratic system of referrals. Administrative inertia within the NHS suggests that this by now well-known problem will not be easily solved, though particular centres of excellence such as Newcastle, East London and Kingston show that where the problem of abortion waiting lists is tackled with energy and imagination, it can be overcome.

One paradox of the long campaign to reform the abortion laws is the recognition by many people that specific abortion legislation is neither necessary nor desirable, any more than it is necessary to legislate specifically for appendicitis or tonsillectomy or any other operation. The abortion notification form is often resented as grossly intrusive, and there are growing doubts expressed in parliament and elsewhere about the confidentiality of abortion information (House of Commons Debates, 1982b). There is little evidence that the mass of abortion statistics routinely collected at the cost of more than £100,000 each year (House of Commons Debates, 1982a) has been put to good use. The supervision of the private abortion sector and the processing of the notification forms costs more than another £150,000 each year (House of Commons Debates, 1982a). Some women, unable to obtain NHS abortions, naturally feel that this money might have been put to better use in improving abortion facilities instead of simply swelling an obstructive abortion bureaucracy. It has, moreover, long been recognised that the abortion notification forms give more information about the attitudes of the doctors than about the condition of the patients (Simms, 1971).

The overwhelming majority of abortion patients request abortion because they have decided, for what they believe to be sound reasons of their own, that they do not wish to have a baby, despite the fact that they have become pregnant. No-one has yet been able to demonstrate that anyone other than the woman herself (for instance, husband, doctor, priest, psychiatrist or social worker) is better qualified or better placed to make this decision for her. The 1967 Abortion Act was a half-way house. It handed the abortion decision to the medical profession. The next stage is to hand this very personal decision to the woman herself. Both public opinion and modern technology are moving towards this outcome, which the Women's Movement in general, and the National Abortion Campaign in particular, has always championed.

In 1975 and again in 1979, National Opinion Polls asked the public whether it thought 'abortion should be made legally available for all who want it?', a position that goes far beyond the Abortion Act. In 1975, 52 per cent agreed with this proposition; in 1979, 56 per cent did so. The proportion who disagreed with abortion-on-request had meanwhile fallen from 34 per cent down to 29 per cent. (NOP, 1975, 1979). Younger people approved of liberal abortion much more than the old, the higher and more educated classes much more than the lower ones, and most interesting of all, there was now little difference according to political party. The proportions of Labour, Conservative and Liberal voters who approved of abortion-on-request were 57 per cent, 58 per cent and 61 per cent respectively, whereas in the past few Conservatives would have supported such a radical position.

Nonetheless the problem of regional inequality in abortion provision which has been evident since the Act was passed, has not diminished. There are now many feminist groups who wish to reduce the amount of discretion the health authorities have in this matter and force all of them to provide a reasonable proportion of abortions in their area under the National Health Service. The Government's Merrison Committee which reported on the National Health Service in 1979, recommended that 75 per cent of all abortions in every area ought to be carried out under the National Health Service (Merrison Committee, 1979). In 1981, a Labour MP, Ms Jo Richardson, made the first attempt in Parliament to legislate for this (House of Commons Debates, 1981). Although this bill failed, it seems likely that further attempts will be made during the 1980s to lay a duty on health authorities to improve abortion services and to reduce the inequality of provision that at present obliges some women to travel long distances for this operation.

Opponents of abortion will continue to attempt to restrict the Abortion Act, in particular to try to reduce the gestation period during which abortion is legal. Even if they succeed, it seems unlikely this would seriously affect the total numbers of legal abortions carried out. It is now widely recognised that if any substantial reduction did occur in the availability of legal abortion, then widespread illegal abortion would take its place. Nowadays very early abortion has become so simple that many women's groups could provide their own facilities and it is doubtful whether governments would welcome bringing prosecutions against them in the present state of public opinion.

In recognition of this, the anti-abortion pressure groups are switching part of their attention from Parliament to the law courts, and from abortion to associated issues of life and death. Nurses are being encouraged to declare that they have conscientious objections to abortion, to refuse to take part in the operation, and to publish evidence of abortion 'irregularities' taking place in their hospitals. Several doctors have been threatened with prosecution for failing to resuscitate abnormal newborn babies, after discussion with the parents. One case, that of Dr Leonard Arthur in 1981, was actually brought to trial. He was accused initially of murder, and then of attempted murder, but the jury refused to convict. This was a blow to the members of the *Life* organisation that had prevailed upon the Director of Public Prosecutions to bring the case.

Although the religious pressure groups may score victories from time to time in individual cases, there is little doubt that the main battle for legal abortion has been fought and won, and what now remains is for the administration of the abortion system to be made more equitable and efficient, until such time as abortions can be self-administered and thereby cease to be a political issue.

7 Who's for Amniocentesis? The Politics of Prenatal Screening

Wendy Farrant

> The antenatal diagnosis of fetal defects is perhaps the greatest advance in perinatal medicine for a generation. (*British Medical Journal*, 1978, p. 1661)
>
> the real tragedy, the real scandal, is that so many handicapped babies are ever born in the first place. . . . We have the technology and the skill to detect almost all serious abnormalities in the early stages of pregnancy. (*Guardian* women's page, Toynbee, 1981, p. 12)
>
> A step nearer the day when *every* baby is born healthy. (*Daily Express*, 1977)

Over the past decade, a rapid development has occurred in techniques and services for the detection of foetal abormality in early pregnancy. As the quotations above illustrate, this development has been heralded by the lay and medical press as a major advance. Consumer organisations have joined doctors and politicians in proclaiming the right of every woman to have access to prenatal screening:

> No-one knows how many mothers would refuse an abortion in the almost certain knowledge that they would bear a spina bifida child, but surely every 'at risk' mother has a right to know and to choose for herself. (*CHC News*, 1978, p. 11)
>
> Every woman should be entitled to it. (Stuart Campbell, Professor of Obstetrics and Gynaecology, quoted in Toynbee, 1981, p. 12)
>
> Unlike the Archbishop who wants to deny individuals the right to make their own moral decisions, I believe these tests must be available so women can decide for themselves. (Keith Hampson, Conservative MP, 1978)

Media discussion about conflict of interests has focused almost exclusively on the small but vociferous sector of the anti-abortion lobby who have incorporated opposition to the developing technology into their campaigns to deny women access to abortion.

The purpose of this chapter is to explore the interests that are served by the development of prenatal screening services, and the potential conflict between these interests and those of women who are requesting or being offered the service. The chapter is based on the premise that, whatever the potential of reproductive technologies might be for advancing the interests of women, such technologies are not necessarily developed with the interests of women primarily in mind; nor are they necessarily applied to further women's interests. The chapter begins by charting the growth of prenatal screening services, and moves on to identify some economic, professional and ideological interests with which the service development can be linked. It then looks at some ways in which these interests have shaped the particular form that services have taken, and highlights the implications in terms of neglect of women's needs and control over women's decision making about prenatal screening and abortion. The concluding section focuses on the wider implications, for women and for people with disabilities, of current developments in prenatal screening.

The chapter draws upon findings from a three-year research study of women's experiences of prenatal screening. The study involved following up a series of women who were undergoing prenatal diagnosis in two Area Health Authorities in inner London and interviewing them, after the outcome of the diagnostic investigation had been determined, about their experiences, attitudes and needs. One hundred and thirty-five (95 per cent) of the women who met the criteria for inclusion in the research series agreed to be interviewed. The women in the research series were representative of the social class and ethnic structure of the population of the study area. Sixty-two of these women (the 'serum AFP screened' group) had undergone further investigations (including amniocentesis in 39 cases) as a result of an abnormal finding on a routine maternal serum alphafetoprotein (AFP) screening test[1] for neural tube defects (spina bifida and anencephaly). The remaining 73 women (the 'high risk' group) had had an amniocentesis[2] on account of an increased risk of foetal abnormality associated with their age or their obstetric or family history. The outcome of the prenatal diagnostic investigation was abnormal for 9 women, 8 of whom decided to terminate the pregnancy. Interviews with women were supplemented by interviews with obstetricians and other health workers, by direct observation of counselling and testing sessions, and by an analysis of local and national policy documents. In order to ascertain the extent to which the policy, practice and attitudes of obstetricians in the study area was representative of the profession as a whole, a questionnaire was mailed to a random sample of consultant obstetricians in England and Wales, 323 (65 per cent) of whom replied.

The growth of prenatal screening services

In this chapter, discussion is confined to the more common, current applications of prenatal diagnostic technology, namely its use in the prenatal detection of chromosome disorders (particularly Down's syndrome) and neural tube defects.

Amniocentesis was first used for prenatal diagnosis of chromosome disorders in 1967, and extended to the prenatal detection of neural tube defects in 1973. Since then there has been a rapid increase in the number of women undergoing diagnostic amniocentesis in early pregnancy, and a significant change in the pattern of service delivery (Polani *et al.* 1976; Polani, 1977; Clinical Genetics Society, 1978; Alberman *et al.* 1979). Initially, prenatal diagnosis was confined mainly to a select group of high risk women who had themselves often initiated the referral because of concern about their increased chance of producing a baby with a severe abnormality. As the service has expanded, there has been an increasing trend for referrals for amniocentesis to be doctor – rather than patient – initiated. A particularly important development has been the introduction of *routine* maternal serum AFP screening for neural tube defects.

The development of routine prenatal screening for neural tube defects can be seen as significant in two ways. Firstly, it has introduced the possibility of extending the potential benefits of prenatal diagnosis to women who are at increased risk of having a baby with a neural tube defect but who have no factor in their obstetric or family history to indicate this. Secondly, it could be regarded as representing an extension into the antenatal period of the interventionist trend in the management of labour and delivery, whereby technological innovations originally introduced for the benefit of high risk women have come to have an impact on the childbearing experiences of an increasing proportion of low risk women (Cartwright, 1979; Graham and Oakley, 1981, Garcia, 1982; Oakley, 1982; Rakusen, 1982a).

In 1977 the first report of the UK Collaborative Study concluded that routine maternal serum AFP screening for neural tube defects could be effectively introduced into existing patterns of antenatal care. By the end of that year the service was being provided by at least one district in 31 of the 98 Area Health Authorities in England and Wales, and by 1979 the number of AHAs which had introduced the service had increased to 46 (Wald *et al.* 1979). The service has continued to expand, so that by 1982 routine AFP screening was being offered in one or more districts of at least two-thirds of the former (i.e. pre-reorganisation of the NHS) Area Health Authorities.[3]

Vested interests

So in whose interest has this rapid development of prenatal screening taken place?

Medical commentators have pointed to an increasing demand for prenatal screening from pregnant women of all ages who have uncomplicated histories (*British Medical Journal*, 1977). There seems little doubt that, in contrast to many other areas of technological innovation in obstetrics, the reaction of women to the development of prenatal diagnostic technology has been favourable. Whatever their feelings about their own personal experience of the procedure, the attitude of women in the research series towards the general idea of prenatal screening was, in the main, extremely positive. This favourable attitude can be related to the fears about foetal abnormality that are commonly voiced by pregnant women (Graham, 1980; Homans, 1982). Such fears in part relate to wider societal values regarding people with disabilities (Mason, 1981; Rakusen, 1984), but they also have a grounding in the social reality of women's role as carer (Graham, 1984b) and the additional strain that handicap imposes on that role (Baldwin and Glendinning, 1983). Women's anxieties about foetal abnormality are also reinforced by current health and social policies that have had the effect of exacerbating mothers' feelings of personal responsibility for the health of their baby (Graham, 1980) and of placing the burden of responsibility for the care of children and adults with disabilities even more firmly upon the shoulders of women in the community (Finch and Groves, 1983).

However, consumer interest is not generally the motivating force behind the development of medical technologies and services (Doyal, 1979; Day, 1982).

Closer examination of the development of prenatal screening services suggests that the expansion of services was stimulated less by consumer demand than by initiatives from government, from interested sectors of the medical profession, and from the medical supply industry.

Government

Government consultative documents published in the mid to late 1970s identified prenatal screening as a priority area for expansion. The rationale for favouring the development of this service at a time of general economic restraint is clearly expressed in *Reducing the Risk: Safer Pregnancy and Childbirth*:

> because caring for the handicapped can impose great burdens on our society the prevention of handicap . . . in addition to its other benefits *may save money*. (emphasis added) (DHSS, 1977a, p. 48)

The consultative document *Prevention and Health: Everybody's Business* (DHSS, 1976a) makes reference to cost benefit analyses, which have concluded that the costs of providing amniocentesis for all expectant mothers over the age of 40 years, and maternal serum AFP screening for all pregnant women, would be more than offset by the economic benefits in terms of savings of expenditure on children and adults with Down's syndrome and spina bifida (Glass, 1976; Hagard and Carter, 1976; Hagard *et al.* 1976; Holterman, 1977).

Following the publication in 1977 of the report of the UK Collaborative Study, the DHSS (1977b) issued a draft consultative circular to Regional Health Authorities and professional bodies, encouraging the introduction of routine screening for neural tube defects into existing patterns of antenatal care, and pointing out that the service would pay for itself in three years.

A Working Group on Screening for Neural Tube Defects (under the chairmanship of Sir Douglas Black) was set up by the Standing Medical Advisory Group to advise the government, in the light of comments on the DHSS draft circular, 'on what guidance might be given to health authorities on the introduction into routine antenatal care of a service to detect neural tube defects' (DHSS, 1979a, p. 1). The report of the working group (hereafter referred to as the Black Report on AFP screening) gave prenatal screening a general stamp of approval, that was subsequently endorsed by other official reports such as the Report of the Royal Commission on the National Health Service (1979) and the Second Report from the Social Services Committee on Perinatal and Neonatal Mortality (House of Commons, 1980).

The medical profession

The main groups amongst the medical profession with an interest in prenatal screening are obstetricians and geneticists. Both specialities were strongly represented within the membership of the DHSS Working Group on Screening for Neural Tube Defects, referred to above, and among those who gave evidence to the Working Group.

The professional interest of *obstetricians* in technological innovation has been analysed in general terms by a number of social scientists (e.g. Richards, 1975; Doyal, 1979). Such authors have located this interest within the mechanistic model of contemporary medical practice and ideology, and have pointed to the central role of obstetric technology in enhancing the status of obstetrics as a speciality and in enabling the medical profession to take control of care during pregnancy and childbirth away from midwives and childbearing women. As the potential for innovation in the management of labour and delivery becomes satiated, and evidence of its lack of effectiveness and iatrogenic effects accumulates (Chard and Richards, 1977), the effort to prevent perinatal mortality and morbidity through technical intervention can be seen to be extending backwards into the antenatal period.

The upsurge of obstetric interest in prenatal screening during the latter half of the 1970s can also be related to more immediate economic concerns, stemming from the DHSS (1976b) consultative document *Priorities for Health and Social Services in England*, which singled out hospital maternity services for reduced expenditure. The government's interest in the economic benefits of prenatal screening, which was being expressed at around the same time as the publication of the priorities document, provided obstetricians with a useful weapon in their defence of maternity services against the cuts.

The Royal College of Obstetricians and Gynaecologists (RCOG) were strongly criticised by enthusiasts from within and outside the medical profession for their cautious response to the government's draft proposal for the introduction of routine screening for neural tube defects into existing patterns of antenatal care. However, in encouraging the DHSS to 'make haste slowly' (*Guardian*, 1978) the RCOG made clear that their commitment to the *principle* of setting up an antenatal screening programme was not in doubt. The RCOG's reservations about the DHSS draft consultative circular were explained in a letter to *The Times*, written by representatives of the College in response to a letter by Keith Hampson, MP. The main objection of the RCOG to the DHSS draft proposal was said to be that:

> the costing estimates were felt to be unrealistic and the whole concept was based upon the assumption that adequate ultrasound facilities and expertise in their use were available throughout the country. (Dewhurst and Scott, 1978)

The College therefore recommended that the Department of Health build up the screening service in areas where it already existed, and extend it to other areas only when they could ensure that the necessary back up facilities and staff could be made available. This is the view that prevailed in the Black Report on AFP screening. The RCOG also used the opportunity of the letter to *The Times* to register the profession's objection to 'political pressure [being] applied to influence clinical judgement'.

The interests of *geneticists* were expressed in the report of a working party of the Clinical Genetics Society (1978), set up in 1976 to consider the demand and facilities available for prenatal diagnosis in the UK and to make recommendations for the improvement of such services. The report provided evidence of the unequal development of prenatal diagnostic services throughout the UK and pointed to the importance of local research interests and resources in shaping the distribution of services. At least part of the prenatal diagnostic work of most of the laboratories surveyed by the working party was being funded from non-NHS sources, with research funds continuing to be used to undertake work that had become entirely service in nature.

The Clinical Genetics Society working party expressed concern about the inadequacy of existing NHS support for prenatal diagnostic work and the effects on the quantity and quality of provision, and recommended:

> That the current makeshift arrangements for prenatal diagnosis in the UK be replaced by a comprehensive service organised on a regional basis with funds designated for the purpose by Regional Health Authorities. (Clinical Genetics Society, 1978, p. 26)

Specific recommendations included the provision of facilities for prenatal diagnosis by amniocentesis to cover approximately eight per cent of all pregnancies, and the introduction as soon as possible of a national programme for the detection of neural tube defects by maternal serum AFP screening. It was proposed that the national service should be closely integrated within a network of Regional Genetic Advisory Centres co-ordinated with the help of a Standing Committee on Genetic Services. The report outlined the range of services, in addition to genetic counselling and prenatal diagnosis, that Regional Genetic Centres would wish to have responsibility for and argued that the establishment of such a network 'would represent a rewarding use of Health Service resources' (Clinical Genetics Society, 1978, p. 23). The function of the proposed Standing Committee on Genetic Services would be to ensure 'that the developing service is steered along the right lines by experts from the various disciplines involved' (Clinical Genetics Society, 1978, p. 26).

The medical supply industry

The report of the Clinical Genetics Society working party also provides some insight into the significance of prenatal screening for a further interest group, namely the medical supply industry, who are in a position to make large profits from what the report identifies as the increasing importance of obstetric ultrasound in prenatal diagnosis. The ultrasound market has been described by the industry as 'among the fastest growing medical instrumentation markets of all time' (Association for Improvements in the Maternity Services, 1983, p. 15). Pharmaceutical companies are also profiting from the supply of proprietary kits for maternal serum AFP estimation. Commercially produced testing kits were being used by approximately half of the laboratories undertaking serum AFP estimation that were surveyed by the Clinical Genetics Society working party, although this practice has been criticised on grounds of the high cost and variable reliability of proprietary kits (Clinical Genetics Society, 1978; National Medical Consultative Committee, 1980).

It is then possible to identify specific economic and professional interests that can be linked to the development of prenatal screening services. In addition, the rapid expansion of services needs to be interpreted in relation to the wider ideological and social control functions of medicine in general and obstetric technology in particular (see, for example, Doyal, 1979; Lewis, 1980; Graham, 1980; Roberts, 1981; Day, 1982; Russell, 1982; Elston and Doyal, 1983). This point will be explored further through examination of the attitudes of obstetricians.

A technological fix

Some striking findings of the survey of consultant obstetricians concerned the general enthusiasm of consultants for prenatal screening, and their optimism about its potential for reducing the population incidence of disability.

Although most consultants expressed some reservations about the technological innovation – mainly regarding the potential iatrogenic effects of amniocentesis – the perceived costs were generally regarded as negligible in relation to the perceived benefits. Eighty-five per cent of respondents considered that, on balance, the potential benefits of a national screening programme for the detection of neural tube defects outweighed the potential problems, and only four per cent considered that the problems outweighed the benefits. The benefits of prenatal screening were described by consultants mainly in terms of the perceived advantages for mothers of being able to avoid the birth of a handicapped child. However, the potential benefits were also perceived as extending beyond the individual woman to society as a whole. Thus two-thirds of respondents to the survey rated 'savings in costs to society of caring for people with disabilities' as an important potential benefit of a national screening programme for the prenatal detection of neural tube defects.

Contrary to the impression given by consultants' responses and by the quotations at the beginning of this chapter, the potential of prenatal screening for 'preventing' disability is in fact extremely limited. As an example of the limitations of current screening programmes, Alberman and Berry (1979) have estimated that if all pregnant women over the age of 40 years received amniocentesis and selective termination where indicated (sic) this would result in only 13 per cent of births with Down's syndrome being averted. Furthermore, Down's syndrome and other prenatally detectable conditions account for only a minority of mentally handicapped children (Chard and Richards, 1977). In theory, prenatal screening has more potential for reducing the population incidence of neural tube defects. In practice, however, the clinical efficiency of maternal serum AFP screening is failing to meet up to expectations (Roberts *et al.* 1983). In some districts with a low population incidence of neural tube defects, the predictive value of AFP screening for detecting neural tube defects has proved to be so disappointing that the screening programme has been discontinued (Standing *et al.* 1981; Seller, 1981).

The potential of prenatal diagnostic technology for detecting foetal abnormality also needs to be weighed against its known and unknown potential for causing foetal damage (Enkin and Chalmers, 1982). The current state of knowledge regarding the hazards of amniocentesis is by no means conclusive. However, a study by the Medical Research Council (1978) estimated that amniocentesis is associated with an increased foetal loss (from miscarriage and perinatal mortality) of about 1.0 to 1.5 per cent and a possible increase of 1.0 to 1.5 per cent in certain types of major infant morbidity, namely unexplained respiratory difficulties at birth and major orthopaedic postural abnormalities. On the basis of the findings from the Medical Research Council, the Black Report on AFP screening summarises, for populations with varying incidences of neural tube defects, the benefits of a prenatal screening programme (in terms of number of births with neural tube defects prevented) compared with the physical costs (in terms of the number of normal foetuses harmed by amniocentesis). The cost-benefit ratio becomes progressively less favourable as the population incidence of neural tube defects decreases. This, together with the fact that around 85 per cent of babies with neural tube defects are either still-born or die within the first year of life, means that in regions with a low incidence of neural tube defects 'it is possible that more unaffected pregnancies may be harmed than handicapped children avoided' (DHSS, 1979a, p. 28).

The importance of social and economic factors in the causation of handicap and disability is well documented (e.g. Humphreys, 1979; Walker, 1980; Townsend and Davidson, 1982). In the case of neural tube defects, for example, St. George (1983) has reviewed the evidence relating the high prevalence of neural tube defects in certain population groups to nutritional deficiencies which, in turn, can be related to the production, processing and distribution of food in advanced capitalist societies. An approach to prevention which attempts to bypass the socio-economic determinants of handicap and its disabling social consequences will never be a panacea. From this point of view, unrealistic expectations about the potential of prenatal screening for reducing the population incidence of disability must be seen as reflecting and perpetuating a dominant ideology that deflects attention from the social production of ill health by reifying health problems and their solutions as technical rather than political issues.

A doctor's right to choose

The media publicity given to the views of the small minority of anti-abortion opponents of prenatal screening is unfortunate in that: firstly it has diverted attention away from the profound social, political and ethical implications of recent trends in prenatal screening that lie outside the more general issue of a woman's choice about abortion; and, secondly, it has given the impression that the opponents of a woman's right to make her own decisions about abortion are all located within the anti-screening camp.

That the latter is clearly not the case, was strikingly demonstrated by the signatories to a parliamentary Early Day Motion tabled by Keith Hampson, at the beginning of 1979, calling for the immediate establishment of a nationwide screening programme for the antenatal detection of neural tube defects. The signatories covered a wide range of the political spectrum and included Rhodes Boyson, John Corrie and a number of well known anti-abortion Roman Catholic MPs. The Early Day Motion on screening was tabled a month before the first reading in the House of Commons of Sir Bernard Braine's Abortion (Amendment) Bill. Of the 117 supporters of the Early Day Motion on antenatal screening who also voted in the first hearing of the Braine Abortion (Amendment) Bill, 43 (i.e. over a third) voted *in favour* of restricting the terms of the 1967 Abortion Act.

The advocates of prenatal screening within the medical profession likewise include some outspoken opponents of a woman's right to abortion on social grounds. Professor Ian Donald, on receiving an award for his pioneering work on the use of ultrasound for the detection of foetal abnormality, commented:

> My innate abhorrence of abortion without scientific or medical indication of the need for it is well known. (Donald, 1982, p. 2)

When viewed in the context of the history of abortion reform, the co-existence of pro-screening attitudes with an opposition to abortion on social grounds is not necessarily contradictory. As discussed in Madeleine Simms' chapter in this collection, the right of a woman to choose abortion has never been recognised by parliament or by the medical profession. Also much of the support for abortion reform has been motivated by eugenic concerns rather than by a desire to enhance individual women's reproductive choices (Greenwood and Young, 1976; Riley, 1981). Given this historical background, and the observation that pressures on the Secretary of State to introduce a national prenatal screening programme coincided with renewed pressures (culminating in the 1979 Corrie Abortion Amendment Bill) to restrict women's choices about abortion, it is important to look more closely at the motives of the supporters of prenatal screening. The following observations are based on in-depth interviews with obstetricians from the study area, and on some findings from the survey of consultant obstetricians in England and Wales.

In terms of their attitudes to abortion for foetal abnormality and abortion for social reasons, and their perception of their own role in the decision-making process, consultant obstetricians could be broadly divided into three categories, which I will refer to as the 'opponents', the 'women's advocates' and the 'medical advocates'.

The 'opponents' were those consultants who were opposed to abortion on any grounds, including foetal abnormality. In keeping with the findings from other surveys (Waite, 1972) the number of consultants who fell into this category was extremely small. Although twenty-seven of the 304 respondents to the survey question about abortion identified themselves as having 'a conscientious objection to termination of pregnancy in virtually all cases', only seven of these consultants (i.e. 2 per cent of the total sample) disagreed with abortion in the case of proven foetal abnormality.

The 'women's advocates' were the small group of 32 consultants (10 per cent of the total sample) who expressed agreement with the statement that 'abortion should be readily available *as a right* to anyone who chooses it'. The policy and practice of these consultants in relation to abortion for both medical and social reasons were governed by the woman's wishes and by the principle (to quote a consultant from the study area) that:

> it is just as wrong to assume a woman would want an abortion as to deny one.

The largest category of (245) consultants – the 'medical advocates' – were distinguished from the 'women's advocates' by their belief that the doctor, rather than the woman, should have the right to make the final decision about abortion. When asked, 'If the development of prenatal diagnostic services were competing for resources with the development of NHS facilities for first trimester abortions, which do you feel should receive the highest priority?' two thirds (18 out of 27) of the 'women's advocates' who responded to the question replied 'first trimester abortions' on the basis of the much larger number of women involved. In contrast, 84 per cent (199 out of 226) of the 'medical advocates' who responded to the question replied 'prenatal diagnosis'. The 'medical advocates' explained their preference for the development of prenatal screening services mainly in terms of their own judgement that foetal abnormality is a more important and deserving indication for termination than the reasons for which women seek first trimester abortions. Their reasoning also reflected the importance that the 'medical advocates' attach to keeping decision making about abortion within medical control, and the moral judgements that they make about women seeking abortions:

> At least (prenatal diagnosis and selective abortion) is in some way selective and under true *medical* control. The other (first trimester abortion) is at the whim of politicians and women's libbers.

> At least it (abortion for foetal abnormality) is genuine . . . I believe that more than 95% of first trimester abortions are being carried out on social grounds and usually in women who did not take contraceptive precautions.

> Women cannot control congenital abnormality. They have the means to prevent the unwanted pregnancy.

In addition, the 'medical advocates'' responses were often implicitly, and at times explicitly, eugenic:

> Foetal abnormalities cost the country a great deal of money. Unwanted babies can be productive members of society.

> If there's no chance of foetal abnormality – if it's purely the mother's choice – then you must think of the rights of the unborn child. . . . but if it's abnormal you must place yourself in its position and ask if you were an abnormal child how you would feel about being born.

> With a grossly overcrowded world, we're in a position now to be selective about which people we want in the world.

> For eugenic reasons. At present facilities are being used to preserve abnormal babies while healthy foetuses are destroyed on a large scale.

Some 'medical advocates' who described themselves as having a conscientious objection to abortion made it clear that their ethical objection was not to 'killing' foetuses *per se*, but rather to 'killing' normal foetuses:

> I personally dislike killing normal, healthy foetuses.

> Aborting normal foetuses is wrong in principle.

The major reservations about prenatal screening expressed by respondents to the survey concerned the inadvertent loss of a normal foetus as a result of either spontaneous abortion following amniocentesis or induced abortion following an incorrect diagnosis of foetal abnormality. Again, the expression of such reservations sometimes carried considerable eugenic overtones:

> Normal foetuses may be aborted and thus society may be losing a valuable human contribution.

> Prenatal diagnosis is a greatly overrated procedure and if practised extensively in its present form, kills a *normal* baby for every abnormal discovered . . . If society *really* wants rid of abnormals it must carry out euthanasia at 40 weeks rather than 20 weeks and thereby avoid trauma and death to *normal* foetuses *in utero*.

The relatively high priority that most consultants attach to foetal abnormality as an indication for abortion is reflected by the relatively late gestational stage at which they are prepared to terminate the pregnancy. Over 80 per cent of respondents said that they would be prepared to terminate a pregnancy at 20 weeks or more if Down's syndrome or spina bifida had been diagnosed, and a substantial minority (including some doctors with a conscientious objection to abortion) said that under such circumstances they would be prepared to terminate the pregnancy beyond the legal limit of 28 weeks. For comparison, consultants were asked to state the latest gestational stage (if any) at which they would be prepared to terminate a pregnancy for the following 'high risk' women requesting abortion for reasons other than foetal abnormality: (a) 'a mother of a child with a severe mental or physical handicap who felt that another child, even if normal, would place too much strain on the family', and (b) 'a 40-year-old mother of a teenage child who felt that she could not cope with caring for a baby at this stage of her life'. Ten per cent of respondents said that they would not be prepared to terminate a pregnancy at *any* stage for the latter indications, and less than ten per cent of respondents said that they would be prepared to terminate the pregnancy at 20 or more weeks.

Conflict of interests

It should be clear from the above discussion that not all supporters of antenatal screening are motivated by a desire to enhance a woman's reproductive choices. Nevertheless, some might argue that the motives underlying the development of prenatal screening services are unimportant, so long as the end results are beneficial. I will now attempt to demonstrate how the vested interests identified above have had a distorting effect on the way in which the service has developed, with adverse consequences both for women undergoing screening and at an ideological level.

Allocation of resources

One distorting effect of vested interests already referred to concerns the role of local research and clinical interests in shaping the distribution of services. Although there has been a concentration of research activity and service development in a few high risk areas, notably South Wales and West Scotland, the general pattern of service distribution – in England at least – bears little relation to need, as measured by congenital abnormality statistics.

North East Thames Region – where the study of women's experiences of prenatal screening was based – was the first Regional Health Authority in the country to fund a regional prenatal screening programme for neural tube defects (along with programmes for the prenatal detection of Down's syndrome and thalassaemia). Yet the incidence of births with neural tube defects in North East Thames Region, as in other parts of South East England, is well below the national average (Rogers and Weatherall, 1976). As has happened elsewhere, the development of prenatal screening in North East Thames Region was originally a research initiative, with the Regional Health Authority then coming under pressure from professionals to take over and extend financial support for the programme. The question of whether the resources allocated to the regional prenatal screening programme might have been deployed in ways that would have been more beneficial to women, is especially pertinent at a time of cutbacks in much more basic services, and in view of the discussion earlier in this chapter regarding the limited 'benefits' of AFP screening in a low risk region in relation to the potential problems.

Neglect of women's needs

The major finding to emerge from the study of women's experiences of prenatal screening was the very different experience of women who had been identified as 'at risk' on the basis of a routine screening test for neural tube defects, compared with women who had realised they were at risk before they were pregnant on account of their age or obstetric history. Although the majority of women from both groups were on balance glad the tests had been available, those who had been identified as at risk on the basis of a routine screening programme found the experience much more distressing (Farrant, 1980a). This difference was partly related to the very different emotional implications of prenatal diagnosis for the two groups of women, but was also related to the more intensive counselling needs of the serum AFP screened group and the failure of the service to provide adequately for these needs (Farrant, 1980b, 1983).

The emotional implications of prenatal screening are largely overlooked by the medical profession and by those involved in the planning of services. Discussion of the costs and benefits of screening is usually couched exclusively in financial or physical terms. Although lip service is paid to the importance of good counselling, this is not reflected in the costing of prenatal screening services, or by research priorities. The North East Thames Region proposal (1979) for a prenatal screening programme, for example, included costings for laboratory staff, secretarial assistance and staff time to cover extra ultrasound sessions, but did not make any financial provision for counselling time. The Black Report on AFP screening emphasised the importance of monitoring the impact of the screening programme, at national and local level, in terms of uptake of services, number of neural tube defect births averted and physical complications of amniocentesis, but did not include any mention of a need to monitor the experiences of women undergoing screening and the quality of the counselling that they are being offered.

Biased counselling

The conflict of interests between providers and users of prenatal screening services is clearly reflected in the counselling process. At all stages of screening, counselling is systematically biased towards encouraging women to take up the tests and to have an abortion if an abnormality is detected, rather than providing women with the information and support they require to make an informed choice and to avoid unnecessary distress. This will be illustrated with reference to the successive stages of decision making about screening for neural tube defects.

(i) *Decision about the initial serum screening test.* Because of the potentially serious implications of an abnormal result on a serum AFP screening test, the Black Report on AFP screening recommended that (contrary to the usual procedure of routine testing of blood during pregnancy):

> women should be given the opportunity to 'opt in' to a serum screening programme for neural tube malformations after a full explanation. (DHSS, 1979a, p. 35)

However, the efforts put into encouraging women to attend for antenatal care in time for screening do not seem to have been matched by efforts to ensure that women are given a choice about screening. In response to the survey of consultant obstetricians, which was conducted several months after the Black Report on AFP screening was published, a quarter of consultants said their policy was to give the screening test routinely without offering women any explanation of its purpose or any choice about whether or not they participated in the screening programme.

(ii) *Decision about amniocentesis.* If a woman is not given any option about entering the screening programme then it is meaningless to claim that she has a choice about amniocentesis, since most women would find it difficult not to resolve the uncertainty generated by a positive serum screening test result. Asked whether they were given a choice about having amniocentesis, a number of serum AFP-screened women replied in such terms as:

> I had a choice in that no one would have *forced* me to have it, but psychologically I did not have any choice in that if I hadn't had it I couldn't have gone through with the pregnancy.

> They put me in such a position that if I'd said no [to amniocentesis] I'd have spent the rest of the pregnancy worrying about it.

Nevertheless, because amniocentesis is an invasive procedure that carries a known risk, the professional ethos is that the test should not be given without the woman's informed consent. In practice, however, my research findings suggest that many women are not receiving the necessary information (about risks and limitations of the test, type of abnormality being tested for, etc.) that is required to make an informed decision about amniocentesis. This can be exemplified by the information women are given about the risks of the procedure.

Of the 112 women (including high risk women) interviewed after they had had an amniocentesis, 28 (24 per cent) were unaware that amniocentesis carried a risk of miscarriage, and 96 (86 per cent) were unaware of any other possible hazards. Of the 16 women who were aware of the possible risks to the newborn infant identified in the Medical Research Council study, 12 had obtained this information from sources other than the medical staff who had counselled them about amniocentesis. It is significant that the four women who *had* been informed by a clinician about possible risks to the newborn infant had all been given this information in an attempt to persuade them to change their minds about wanting the test. These four women had all requested amniocentesis on account of their age, but they were all a few years younger than 40 years – the age at which these particular clinicians generally recommend amniocentesis.

The limited information that women in the research series received about the possible hazards of amniocentesis was consistent with advice about counselling contained in the Black Report on AFP screening, and with the policy of most respondents to the survey of consultant obstetricians.

As mentioned earlier, the current stage of knowledge regarding the risks of amniocentesis is by no means conclusive. Nevertheless, the

Black Report on AFP screening took the possible hazards identified by the MRC study sufficiently seriously to recommend that:

> in cases in which amniocentesis has been performed and in which no fetal abnormality has been detected, *the baby should be supervised for possible respiratory difficulties at birth and examined within a few days for orthopaedic postural deformities which may require early treatment, and at intervals until walking is established.* (emphasis added) (DHSS, 1979a, p. 43)

The Black Report's advice just cited, on screening newborn babies for possible effects of amniocentesis, contrasts markedly with the 'Counselling' section of the Report, which recommends informing women only 'that the amniocentesis carries a small risk of miscarriage' (DHSS, 1979a, p. 35)

Of the 304 consultants who replied to the survey question about counselling regarding the hazards of amniocentesis, 96 per cent said that the possible increased risk of miscarriage should generally be discussed with a woman who is offered amniocentesis. However, less than 20 per cent of consultants considered it appropriate to discuss with the woman the possible risks to the newborn infant identified in the MRC report, and only 39 per cent considered it appropriate to discuss 'the uncertainty of the present state of knowledge regarding the hazards of amniocentesis'.

A possible reason for singling out the risk of miscarriage from all the other possible hazards women could be warned about, might be that if a woman has a miscarriage within a few days of having an amniocentesis then there is going to be no doubt in anyone's mind about the causal connection. Certainly the *way* in which women in the research series were informed about the risk of miscarriage, often suggested more concern with avoiding the medico-legal risk of withholding this information than with enabling the woman to make a considered decision. The woman quoted below is labelled in her case-notes as having 'refused' amniocentesis recommended as a result of an abnormal serum screening test result:

> From what the first doctor said it [amniocentesis] seemed a straightforward thing. I'm not medically experienced so I don't know what to ask or what to think of their advice. I've never heard of alpha protein. I just thought they know what they're doing so I'd leave it up to them. I was given the option of having the test, but he said it would be for the best or something so I automatically said 'yes'. It was when I went to have it [amniocentesis] a week or two later that I was told about the risk. He'd prepared me to do it and was just about to stick the needle in when he told me I could go into labour. It scared the life out of

> me because I wasn't prepared for it. He was very abrupt when I said I wanted to think about it . . . [but] I wanted to talk it over with my husband. I didn't want to be rushed into something I didn't know nothing about.

The concept of 'choice' about amniocentesis also needs to be located within the context of antenatal care which generally provides women with very little control over decisions about their own treatment (Graham and Oakley, 1981). Although most (but by no means all) women who were offered amniocentesis understood they had a choice, the majority also felt that a decision not to have the test would have met with medical disapproval:

> She said it's up to you but I got the impression that if I didn't have the test done they wouldn't have cared for me so much as a patient.

> I was booked in for amniocentesis before I'd been consulted about it . . . They said they must ask your permission but they assumed you'd say yes.

> They said you don't have to have the test but it's the rules when you're over 40 (years of age).

The most extreme examples of lack of information concerned black and working class women. Five of the ten non-English-speaking women in the research series had undergone amniocentesis without having any idea about the purpose, potential hazards, or results of the investigation.

(iii) *Decision about termination of pregnancy.* One policy highlighting the difference in perspective between providers and users of prenatal screening services, is the requirement that an amniocentesis should be given only on the condition that the woman first agrees, at least provisionally, to have a termination of pregnancy should the result be abnormal. Three-quarters of respondents to the survey of consultant obstetricians said they generally require women to agree to termination of an affected pregnancy before proceeding to amniocentesis. This policy reflects the medical and administrative view that the whole purpose of prenatal screening is the abortion of an abnormal foetus, and if the woman is not going to agree to an abortion then it is a waste of resources. As one obstetrician put it:

> It's a waste of money if she's not going to act on the information.

When asked what their response would be to a request for amniocentesis from 'a 42 year old mother of a child with Down's syndrome, who was firmly opposed to the idea of abortion but had nevertheless decided that she would like to know in advance whether her next child was going to be a mongol', over half of the consultants said that they would refuse to agree to the request.

The option to abort an affected foetus was also an important potential benefit perceived by women undergoing amniocentesis. However, it was by no means the only perceived benefit, nor was it always the main one.

A major reason for undergoing amniocentesis cited by high risk women was to obtain the reassurance of a negative result – an outcome that is statistically much more likely than a diagnosis of foetal abnormality. The relative lack of importance consultants attach to the woman's need for reassurance is reflected in their policy and practice regarding the communication of a negative result. Whereas 80 per cent of respondents to the survey of consultant obstetricians rated the communication of a *positive* result on amniocentesis as 'very urgent', only 23 per cent rated the communication of a *negative* result as 'very urgent'. A quarter of consultants said that they usually waited until the next routine antenatal appointment to inform the woman of a negative amniocentesis result, and a few said that they did not usually report the result at all if it was negative.

Another potential benefit, mentioned spontaneously by over a third of the women interviewed, was the opportunity to prepare for the birth of a handicapped baby in the case of the mother not wishing to have an abortion. Although most women (77 per cent) had provisionally decided in favour of an abortion for the main type of foetal abnormality they were being tested for, 90 per cent of women could name *some* type of abnormality for which they would not choose to have an abortion. The majority of women said they would still like to know about the abnormality in the latter case, in order to prepare themselves for the birth. This was also the view of a small but significant minority of six women who underwent amniocentesis knowing that they would definitely not want an abortion if the result was abnormal. It was also the reason for the positive attitude towards prenatal screening of the one woman who – following a long and difficult decision-making process – decided to continue with her pregnancy after open spina bifida had been diagnosed.

The policy of offering amniocentesis only on condition that the woman first agrees to abortion of an affected foetus, ignores the needs of the small group of women just referred to. It also reveals a failure to comprehend the complexity of the decision about termination of pregnancy, and the ambivalence experienced even by women who had provisionally decided they would want a termination.

Although all the women had reflected on the possibility of having the pregnancy terminated, a fifth were still undecided, at the time when the final results came through, about what they would have done if the diagnosis had been positive. Others emphasised that although they had provisionally decided that they would (or in a few cases would not) have an abortion, it was impossible to predict how they would have reacted if actually faced with the decision. Sixty-eight per cent of high risk women and 88 per cent of AFP-screened women felt the decision about termination of pregnancy was better left until after the final diagnostic result, partly because it was impossible to make a final decision in the absence of more information about such facts as the nature and implications of the abnormality diagnosed. They also did not want to dwell too much on the possibility of abortion before it was really necessary. The serum AFP-screened women in particular, expressed a need to 'take things one step at a time' and to try and remain optimistic about the pregnancy. The requirement to make a premature decision on the basis of insufficient information was therefore extremely distressing:

> I wasn't sure that I wanted to decide about termination of pregnancy then . . . I felt he was anticipating the results too soon. They have to make you aware of the *possibility* of abortion but I didn't feel you should be expected to make a decision then . . . For the 9 out of 10 who turn out normal I felt it caused *unnecessary* distress . . . It was put to me to decide, but I was not given adequate information or counselling. I was just given the medical facts. If the results were abnormal I would want to seek paediatric advice about the prognosis and *then* decide about termination.

The policy of requiring a decision about abortion prior to amniocentesis, also acts as an indirect and direct source of pressure on the decision making of the small minority of women who end up with a diagnosis of foetal abnormality:

> I felt the way it was put to me if I had the test I would lose the baby if something was wrong. He said that they only agree to do the fluid test if you're prepared to lose the child if it has spina bifida.

One woman, on expressing her ambivalence about abortion of a foetus with Down's syndrome, was reminded by the consultant of the decision that she had made before amniocentesis:

> He talked to me and said 'nothing has changed – you'd already made a decision before you knew [the result] and the situation is still the same'. He said 'you did tell me your husband had said he

couldn't go through with another handicapped child and you said you would have it terminated'. I agreed that I'd said that but . . . .

Although the professional ethos is that women should make their own decisions about termination of pregnancy, the underlying assumption is often that the decision to enter a screening programme is tantamount to a decision to have an abortion if an abnormality is detected. Thus one of the model explanatory leaflets appendaged to the Black Report on AFP screening includes the sentence:

> If for any reason you and your husband would find a termination of pregnancy unacceptable, we suggest not testing a sample of blood for the purposes of detecting a neural tube defect. (DHSS, 1979a, p. 37)

The Black Report on AFP screening bases its costing of a screening programme on the assumption that a proportion of women will choose not to have the initial blood test, but makes no allowance for women subsequently choosing not to have a termination of pregnancy. The Report also talks about the need for 'pre- and post-termination' counselling, but makes no mention of a possible need for counselling following a decision *not* to have a termination of pregnancy.

Of the nine women interviewed after termination of pregnancy, or (in one case) after the decision to continue with the pregnancy following a prenatal diagnosis of spina bifida, only one woman felt that the pros and cons of termination of pregnancy had been fully discussed. The other eight women – irrespective of their final decision about termination of pregnancy, or the ease or difficulty of arriving at that decision – all said that they would have found the experience less distressing if they had been offered more information and/or more opportunity for discussion:

> It's your decision but you don't know *why* you're having it taken away – what's wrong with it – until you talk about it . . . There are so many things you've got to think of before you make up your mind to have it taken away . . . They should have somewhere for you to go and talk to someone with time to talk to you – not a doctor with other patients to see . . . and they should have a place where people carrying a spina bifida can go and see what they are like.

Although all of these eight women were aware that the decision about termination of pregnancy was ultimately their own, it was also made clear to them what the 'sensible' decision would be:

> The decision was made by the doctors. They said 'It's no use, the

tests show it's abnormal. It's up to you what you do, but if you keep it you will live with the problem'.

The double standard applied by some doctors in their counselling of women about abortion for foetal abnormality, compared with abortion for other statutory indications, is illustrated by the following example. This (AFP-screened) woman was faced with an extremely distressing experience of termination of pregnancy for foetal abnormality at five months, after being refused an earlier abortion that she had requested on medico-social grounds:

> [the gynaecologist] didn't really want to do it [abortion for medico-social reasons] . . . He kept saying you're young and healthy, you can cope . . . He said you'll be risking your life and everything having it at four months, so I had to accept it . . . They shouldn't try to talk you out of something you really want in the beginning . . . They try to push you into getting rid of it when there's something wrong with it – they keep saying it's best for you and this and that.

Conclusion

For women, the development of prenatal screening, like other types of reproductive technology (Elston and Doyal, 1983; Roberts, 1984) has been contradictory. In the context of a society which devalues people with disabilities and holds mothers to be responsible both for the prevention of congenital abnormality and for the care of children who are born with disabilities, women have looked to prenatal screening as a means of allaying fears about foetal abnormality and of gaining some control over the possibility of producing a baby with a severe handicap. For certain high risk women, the technical potential of prenatal screening for enhancing a woman's reproductive choices and for making pregnancy a more carefree experience is a real one. However, because prenatal screening has not been developed with the interests of women primarily in mind, it often fails to take account of women's needs, and it has also increased the potential for others to control women's reproduction. Also for many women – particularly low risk women – prenatal screening has become yet another way in which medical care detracts from the possibility of pregnancy being experienced as a normal and enjoyable event.

Furthermore, far from relieving the responsibility that is placed on mothers, prenatal screening can be seen as feeding into and reinforcing a dominant ideology that poses solutions to disability in terms of medical science and maternal responsibility, rather than social and political change.

To quote a 40 year old woman in the research series, who agreed to amniocentesis only after considerable pressure from medical staff:

> It puts a lot of onus on your responsibility. If the mother doesn't know about it [foetal abnormality] she can't be blamed for going through with it [the pregnancy] . . . It's O.K. for the hospital doing experiments, and it's probably for the good of humanity, but that doesn't always help the mother in that situation. It's a sort of blackmail, isn't it? If you don't have it [amniocentesis] and you have a mongol you blame yourself, and if you have it and lose the baby [through miscarriage caused by amniocentesis] you blame yourself.

The possibility of women being blamed for their decisions about prenatal screening and selective abortion became a reality for the woman who decided to continue with her pregnancy following a prenatal diagnosis of spina bifida:

> Every time there was a knock at the door or a letter we thought 'here's another lecture'. They kept saying things like it was wrong to keep the baby . . . it would be wicked . . . They meant well but . . .

In addition to the implications for individual pregnant women, it is important to consider the wider societal implications of the way in which prenatal screening services are being introduced. As discussed earlier, the potential of prenatal screening for reducing the population incidence of disability is very limited. In this context it was disturbing to hear women in the research series expressing the following views about recent trends in prenatal screening:

> It's a fantastic thing . . . How come there's so many abnormal children? Why aren't more tests done?

> I think it should be done on everyone. They shouldn't be brought into the world these children.

> I think people should have it without asking them. . . In a few years there won't be abnormal babies.

Such attitudes are reflective of and reinforced by the sort of media publicity referred to in the introduction to this chapter, by the cost effective arguments being used to support the development of prenatal screening services, and by current preventative health policies that emphasise increased uptake of antenatal services as a solution to perinatal morbidity. Discussion of the longer term implications of current trends in prenatal screening is outside the scope of this chapter, but the effects of fostering the type of beliefs expressed above could clearly be far reaching – including reduced tolerance of disability, further diversion of resources away from the care of people with disabilities and from more socially-oriented approaches to prevention, social censure of women who choose not to be screened, and pressures towards non-voluntary screening.

The eugenic implications of the ideology that underlies and is perpetuated by current developments in prenatal screening has been the subject of recent discussion by members of the Liberation Network for People with Disabilities in this country (Mason, 1982) and the disability rights movement in the United States (Finger, 1984; Saxton, 1984). Such implications have been vehemently denied by the parliamentary and medical advocates of prenatal screening. Keith Hampson, for example, writing in the *Guardian*, argued:

> . . . no one is suggesting that any pregnant woman should be forced to have these tests. Every stage is voluntary. It is not social engineering. (Hampson, 1978)

However, as we have seen in the preceding discussion of 'biased counselling', the distinction between voluntary and non-voluntary screening is not always that clear-cut. Also, while the current professional ethos is for expectant parents to make their own decisions about amniocentesis and selective abortion, the possibility of non-voluntary screening is not totally discounted. To quote some leading geneticists:

> it seems to us inevitable for practical reasons that society will gradually take a more active role in encouraging abortion for these severe untreatable conditions. (Littlefield *et al.* 1973, p. 49)

Forty-one (13 per cent) of the respondents to the survey of consultant obstetricians expressed agreement with the statement that, 'The state should not be expected to pay for the specialised care of a child with a severe handicap in cases where the parents had declined the offer of prenatal diagnosis of the handicap'.

These issues receive little, if any, attention in the lay and medical press or in government reports, which tend to see prenatal screening as presenting an ethical dilemma only for women with a religious objection to abortion. In response to the question, 'What, if any, do you see as the potential hazards to *society* of recent developments in the prenatal detection of foetal abnormality?' the most common response of respondents to the survey of consultant obstetricians was 'none'.

In fact, as was the case with consultant obstetricians, religion was found to be relatively unimportant in determining women's views about prenatal screening. As one Roman Catholic woman put it, 'Religion doesn't come into it when there's handicap involved'. The greatest moral anguish was expressed not by the women with a religious objection to abortion on social grounds, but rather by two teachers of handicapped children, who were conscious of a contradiction between the ideology of prenatal screening and their personal values regarding the position in society of people with disabilities. For instance:

> It was all very well thinking about it from the outside, but quite different when it becomes a personal thing . . . The question of almost loyalty to my former pupils came up, especially the mongols. Because of my work with mental handicap I felt that they should have a position in society too, and if they don't then there's something wrong with society, not them.

In focusing on some potential problems of recent developments in prenatal screening, I do not wish to undermine what many women – particularly high risk women – see as its very real benefits, or to detract from the need for more resources so that these benefits can be more equally distributed. Neither do I wish to detract attention from the deplorable actions of those anti-abortionists who are attempting to deny women access to the technology. I would argue, however, that the greatest threat to a woman's right to choose about prenatal screening and selective abortion comes not from the opponents of prenatal screening, but rather from its advocates. Not only are the opponents of prenatal screening few in number, but there is a powerful parliamentary and medical lobby to curb their influence. The Clinical Genetics Society, for example, notes:

> Some medical practitioners, in order merely to avoid future recriminations, briefly mention to mothers at risk the possibility of amniocentesis without adequate explanation; others, who for non-professional reasons actively discourage consideration of amniocentesis, fail to indicate that she is entitled to a second opinion; both practices are to be deprecated. (Clinical Genetics Society, 1978, p. 14)

There is no such attempt to deprecate the much more prevalent practices referred to in this chapter of, for example, screening without the woman's informed consent or offering amniocentesis only on the condition that the woman first agrees to abortion of an affected foetus.

Also, as is the case for any type of reproductive technology, a woman's right to choose about prenatal screening involves much more than access to the technology and the freedom to make our own decisions. At the very least it implies access to information on which to base our decisions – including information about the meaning of disability that is based on the experiences and perspective of disabled people and mothers of disabled children, rather than on the social stereotypes, fears and prejudices about disability that we ourselves have internalised (Mason, 1981; Hearn, 1983; Rakusen, 1984). The right to choose also implies much more fundamental changes in those aspects of the social, economic and political organisation of our society that result in the marginalisation of women and of people with disabilities, and which structure women's choices about prenatal screening.

Notes

1. *Maternal serum AFP screening for neural tube defects* involves offering a special blood test – alphafetoprotein (AFP) test – to all expectant mothers between the sixteenth and the eighteenth week of pregnancy. If the AFP level is higher than the normal cut-off point (usually taken as 2.5 times the median) for the gestational age, the blood test is usually repeated and an ultrasound examination is carried out. If the second blood test result is also high and the scan does not provide any explanation for the positive blood test result (e.g. multiple pregnancy, or incorrect estimation of gestational age) then amniocentesis is offered. If the AFP concentration of the amniotic fluid is above the normal limit, the woman is offered a termination of pregnancy.
2. *Amniocentesis*, for the diagnosis of foetal abnormality, is usually performed between the sixteenth and eighteenth week of pregnancy. It involves inserting a needle through the abdominal wall into the uterus and drawing off a sample of amniotic fluid. Chromosome abnormalities are diagnosed by growing and examining the foetal cells which are contained in the fluid, and neural tube defects by measuring the concentration of alpha-fetoprotein (AFP) which is raised in the presence of neural tube defects and certain other types of foetal abnormality.
3. Derived from data presented in the Maternity Alliance (1982) survey of antenatal screening provided by district health authorities.

Acknowledgements

The research on which this chapter is based was carried out at the Institute for Social Studies in Medical Care, and supported by a grant from the National Fund for Research into Crippling Diseases. The views expressed in this chapter are mine and do not necessarily represent the views of the Institute or of the funding body.

I am indebted to the women in the research series and the obstetricians, all of whom so generously gave their time to share their views and experiences of prenatal screening.

I would also like to thank the many friends and colleagues who provided support, encouragement and help during the process of developing the ideas contained in this chapter, and who commented on various drafts. In particular, I would like to express my special thanks to Mary Ann Elson, Hilary Graham, Hilary Homans, Maj Hulten, Micheline Mason, Naomi Pfeffer, Jill Rakusen and Jill Russell.

8 By Design: Reproductive Strategies and the Meaning of Motherhood

Ellen Lewin

This chapter presents what I believe to be a somewhat novel perspective on the meaning of motherhood in women's lives. I view women not as passive recipients of circumstance, but as active strategists who create a resource for themselves in the course of becoming and being mothers. Using material I have collected over the past ten years, I will show how women can use both traditional and alternative health care systems, methods and approaches in their strategic quest. The particular goals women seek to maximise are culturally and situationally specific, and the consciousness which accompanies the pursuit of these goals may vary tremendously. The examples I will present illustrate both how motherhood itself may be used strategically and how women may select alternative methods of becoming mothers and interacting with the health care system in ways which permit them to optimise valued objectives. An exhaustive review of the varied experiences of women who become mothers outside conventional family circumstances cannot be attempted here; the case material is intended to illustrate wider issues rather than be descriptive of 'typical' experience.

During the past decade, feminist anthropologists have undertaken research on women in a variety of cultural contexts and have produced impressive evidence of the ways in which gender as a cultural construct articulates with other social and cultural factors. Despite this awareness of cross-cultural diversity, however, the anthropology of gender has tended to rest on an implicit assumption that motherhood is consistently central in the lives of women and that its universal attributes can be understood to account for other features of women's role and status. Motherhood has been seen by some as the limiting condition of the division of labour by sex; Judith Brown, for example, in an early and still influential paper (1970), concluded her cross-cultural survey of women's roles in production by characterising women's work as that which is compatible with child-rearing activities. In her formulation, and those of others who have used cross-cultural comparison to derive minimally common features of sex roles, maternal functions come first, and along with the wider environment, must be adapted to.

Using a different theoretical perspective, Sherry Ortner, in a controversial and influential paper, 'Is Female to Male as Nature is to Culture?' (1974), pointed to woman's reproductive capacity as being at the heart of her identification in all (or nearly all) cultural settings with the devalued domain of 'nature'; in particular, it is women's life-giving functions which mark her, as women are seen to mediate between the human and the natural. Along the same lines, Nancy Chodorow (1974) explicitly pointed to motherhood as the defining feature of the female experience. Woman's status, in her view, derives from her specialisation in mothering; her continuing activity in this domain is motivated in Chodorow's view by the inexorable dynamic of the mother–daughter tie, which overrides any tendency women might have to attempt to avoid motherhood and its attendant social disadvantages. On yet another front, Rosaldo (1974), proposed that women and men divide the social world into domestic and public arenas respectively, and that the domestic setting is largely defined by the maternal tasks of child-rearing which take place there. Fatherhood, in contrast, is understood to occur conceptually at another level; while rights in children – paternity – as mediated by the intricacies of kinship systems, may provide societies with their basic social structural features, fatherhood is rarely seen to be as defining of men as motherhood seems to be of women.

On yet another front, Marxist anthropologists have also looked to motherhood as a basic framework to describe women's social and economic situation. In this varied body of work, women's role in the sexual division of labour has been viewed in terms of the work they do in reproducing the work force, that is in bearing, caring for and socialising children. Their roles in other economic arenas, notably that of production, are arrayed around their reproductive functions, which sometimes are seen in these approaches as work and which are understood, in turn, to determine the conditions under which women may participate in other economic domains (see Edholm, *et al.* 1977, for a recent critique of Marxist thinking in this area).

Despite the diverse aims of the anthropological perspectives mentioned, a common thread unites them. When motherhood is understood to be prior to everything else, to be the essential condition against which other dimensions of the female experience are arranged, it becomes an environmental factor to which women must adapt. From a biological perspective it limits women's physical potential; from a social perspective it limits how they organise their behaviour; from a cultural perspective it limits how they are perceived. The work of motherhood not only limits the extra-domestic, but also the extra-maternal work that women engage in. The meanings attached to motherhood and reproduction are thus seen as limiting definitions of women's value.

The perspective I wish to present here involves a somewhat different emphasis from that which has been discussed so far; it constitutes an alternative insofar as it suggests a more dynamic approach, which brings us closer to an understanding of how women operate strategically in the world.

My approach requires that we look at motherhood not only as a condition to which an adaptation must be made, but as a *resource*, primarily insofar as it enhances the solidification of key affiliative ties and permits women to pursue a variety of aims. In particular, maternal strategies may be considered as an adaptation to compromised social status and to cultural devaluation.

Despite their increasing participation in the work force, women remain segregated in the lowest-paid and least rewarding domains of employment; this not only means that women have little economic power, but that they experience few opportunities for achievement, accomplishment and gratification in the public domain. This occurs at the same time that popular ideology promotes the importance of achievement as a goal for women and that the structure of social relations makes men (and their accomplishments) a primary reference group for women.

I view the seeking out of motherhood not as the expression of inexorable biological forces, but as a demonstration of a particular kind of adaptation to adversity, as behaviour which may be said to be *rational*. I believe that this approach to motherhood also makes the decision *not* to become a mother (which must be dealt with in some other forum) comprehensible as more than deviance or mishap. While accidents do, of course, characterise some aspects of individuals' progress through life, from a socio-cultural vantage point they merge with other, more purposeful, behaviour. In viewing women's behaviour as strategic, I follow Whitten and Whitten (1972, p. 255) who define a strategy as a pattern formed by the many separate, specific behaviours people devise to attain and use resources and to solve the immediate problems confronting them. A strategy is in this sense a choice made by an individual, not necessarily consciously, between various options or competing ways of achieving satisfaction with respect to some external or internal exigency or constraint. Strategic actors are not necessarily in possession of all information needed to make the 'best' decision; often they 'make do' with imperfect alternatives, or select a course of action in the absence of sufficient data. Nor does the interpretation of rationality imply full intentionality; rather, the notion that women act in strategic or rational ways in organising their behaviour serves to express by way of analogy the belief that women's behaviour, like that of other humans, is created in constant interaction with biological, social and cultural constraints, and that outcomes in any and all of these domains may be interpreted to represent a dynamically adaptive process.

The strategies revealed in women's efforts to become mothers are not only situationally specific, in that they provide a response to particular material and social conditions, but are embedded in particular cultural patterns. Among the Latin American immigrants I studied in San Francisco a decade ago (Lewin, 1974; Browner and Lewin, 1982), for example, motherhood was a goal that had meaning at two levels. First, it was used more or less explicitly to create long term solidary ties with offspring which were seen as the source both of immediate personal welfare and of future affiliation. Ties with husbands were not expected to be of long duration (although they often were) both because of notions about the fundamental differences between masculine and feminine motivations and because of the actual observations women had made of the uncertainty of relationships with men. In fact, the formation of a 'family' consisting of mother and children was such a high priority that marriage itself was largely defined as a means to attaining this end.

Central to maternal strategies in this context is a notion of reciprocity. Motherly services are seen as engendering loyalty and strong affective ties, and in this sense imply a potential exchange, however distant its eventual consummation. Although the links between mother and child, the dyadic contracts (Foster, 1961, 1963) that are established between them, begin as vertical ties between people of unequal status, the thrust of this inequality changes over time as the child is transformed from the recipient of services to their provider. From this perspective, it might be said that it is the dynamic quality of this relationship, its continuity and lack of final resolution, that provides its motivating force.

In seeking to solidify children's loyalty, the San Francisco Latinas I studied explicitly manipulated images of maternal altruism and self-sacrifice at the same time that they attempted to exert control over children's activities. Everything in the environment of these Latin American immigrant women forced them to base their long term economic and affiliative strategies on motherhood. While having children soon after marriage initially served as a strategy for strengthening the conjugal bond, having a child functioned as a second line of defence against material deprivation and emotional isolation, especially vital for immigrants whose other social ties are subject to disruption and insecurity and who lack direct access to the economic market place. Claims to maternal 'goodness', then, advanced women's rights to future loyalty; as one informant said, 'If your children know what you've given up for them, they'll always do what you ask'.

In this aspect, Latinas' maternal strategies bear a striking resemblance to the behaviours Margery Wolf observed among Chinese women in Taiwan (1972). Although the informal family units women create, which Wolf calls 'uterine families', lack the enduring qualities of father-centred patrilineages, they serve the affiliative needs of women during their lifetimes. While they have no jural or social structural reality, uterine families are affectively substantial and offer means for furthering women's aims in the many domains of Chinese culture in which they have no sanctioned role.

At a second level of significance, Latinas' maternal strategies articulated in clear ways with the well-established ideology of marian purity, of maternal altruism and self-sacrifice. From this perspective, we may view the ideology as offering a cultural framework within which personal goals could be pursued and which gave meaning and value to the pursuit of these goals. But ideology is not a blueprint which women (or men, for that matter) slavishly follow. Under other sorts of social and economic conditions, in situations in which links with children do not constitute pathways to economic security or personal influence, the maternal strategy may be de-emphasised, and while marian altruism may continue to have some prominence as abstract philosophy, a different dimension of the larger feminine role complex may achieve greater salience (Browner and Lewin, 1982).

Affiliation is not the only 'good' which women seek to maximise through motherhood, for motherhood may also be seen as a primary means of achieving a satisfying identity. In American culture, central value is placed on the individual. As Dumont explains it:

> This individual is quasi-sacred, absolute; there is nothing over and above his legitimate demands; his rights are limited only by the identical rights of other individuals. (Dumont, 1970, p. 4)

The formation of a satisfying and satisfactory personal identity is an explicitly sought after goal. The prevalent notion is that personal identity is to be *achieved* rather than ascribed. To use contemporary jargon, American culture teaches us that we are capable of 'self-actualisation' and that reaching a meaningful individual identity is a central task for each person, regardless of sex.

Data on single mothers, gathered during a study I began in 1977, provide some striking illustrations of the intersection between valued aspects of identity and motherhood in our culture. Roughly equal subsamples of lesbian and heterosexual women, including both 80 formerly married mothers and 56 women who had had children outside of marital situations, were interviewed in the course of the research, which focused on the structure of mothers' social networks and their mobilisation in times of need. Particularly useful in the present discussion are the comments of intentional single mothers, women who consciously decided to become mothers and who followed a course of planned action leading to pregnancy or adoption. Among those interviewed were 31 lesbians, about half of whom, from the perspective I am using here, may be considered the most purposeful in their drive to become mothers. For women who do not under ordinary circumstances interact sexually with men, pregnancy is unlikely to occur accidentally or as the result of a strategy for gaining an affiliation with a man. Data collected on these women offer a unique opportunity for examining maternal strategies in what might be considered an uncontaminated context and to separate meanings attached to motherhood from the usually related issues of marriage and conventional family organisation.

The fact that both lesbian and heterosexual intentional mothers described becoming a mother in terms of the achievement of a valued identity corroborates the view that American culture is concerned with the fulfilment of the individual. Achieving a satisfying identity may involve both a sense of being a 'good' or productive person or experiencing the accomplishment of something important and meaningful beyond the moment. As one intentional single mother said when asked about the meaning of being a mother,

> You get to have a lot of input in another human being's very formative years. That's real special to have that privilege of doing that, and you get to see them growing and developing and it's sort of like you put in the fertile soil and . . . hopefully what will happen is that they grow and blossom and become wonderful . . . I think it's definitely the most important thing that people do . . . to build the next generation.

In a somewhat different vein, a lesbian mother whose child had been born through artificial insemination said that having a child presented her with an opportunity to do battle against what she viewed as a depressed, negative view of life:

> That's why I felt like I wanted to have a kid, because I felt like I could share my joy, and then maybe there would be another joyful person.

Taking a more personal perspective, another lesbian mother described her feelings about motherhood in terms of its effect on her as a person. She sees children as more 'honest' than adults and contact with children, therefore, as a source of both moral improvement and emotional freedom:

> Somehow [having a child] freed me . . . It was like a freeing process for me. The stuff that everybody bottles up, you can let go around kids . . . It was like a re-education . . . It helps me a lot, I

> mean it helps me in everything I do. It helps me see the world better. It helps me feel other people better. It helps me, you know, understand what's happening with the people I work around and all these different things . . . I'm not sure how I figured out that having kids was going to do that for me. Obviously it is a selfish motive, but my life felt really icy without them. I mean inside of me felt kind of devoid of emotion.

Similarly, another lesbian mother said that motherhood has:

> made me more accepting of people who have made different decisions than I did. I used to be a lot more judgemental . . . Now I can more see that people do seem to do things from their own loving perspective . . .

Like many other intentional single mothers I interviewed, motherhood provided the occasion for a woman to declare her commitment to a kind of authenticity, a naturalness, that motherhood connotes. Beyond this, these mothers, like formerly-married women I studied, and in common with other research findings on women's postpartum experience (Hoffman, 1978; Entwistle and Doering, 1981), saw becoming a mother as an event which allowed them to achieve adulthood and womanhood and established them firmly as members of families. The creation of family ties proceeded both because the mother and her child constituted a new family and because having a child tended to bring her into closer alliance with her family of origin.

Strategies for using artificial insemination

Women not only pursue valued goals by being mothers, but may also act strategically in the course of becoming pregnant. Using the example of artificial insemination by donor, I will suggest some ways in which women's personal strategies intersect with their use of the health care system, creating a variety of pathways for accomplishing the same final objective. The cases I will discuss specifically illustrate the ways in which women seek to enhance either autonomy vis-à-vis the health care system, or anonymity vis-à-vis the biological father at the same time that they attempt to become mothers.

Before presenting this material, I'd like to begin with some general background on artificial insemination and its use in human reproduction. The procedure was originally developed for use in animal husbandry, and was first applied to human impregnation in the nineteenth century (Finegold, 1964, p. 7). While early practice concentrated on using husbands' sperm for insemination of their wives, it took little time for the utility of the procedure for wives of sterile husbands to be noted and for interest in artificial insemination by donor (AID) to quicken. By the early years of the twentieth century, the procedure was being employed with some frequency for otherwise infertile couples. Male control over AID was strictly maintained: wives could not be inseminated without their husbands' consent, and debate raged over whether AID might constitute a type of adultery. As recently as 1979 (Ledward, Crawford and Symonds, 1979), debate continued in Great Britain over the propriety of extending legitimacy to children born through AID, a principal argument being that the birth of such offspring did not represent continuation of the bloodline. The practice has also been condemned on religious grounds because it involves commission of the twin sins of adultery and masturbation. Despite these concerns, and the wide variety of strong emotional reactions which the procedure stimulates, AID conceptions are far from rare, possibly accounting for between 6,000 and 10,000 births each year in the United States (Curie-Cohen, Luttrell and Shapiro, 1979, p. 588).

AID, managed through sperm banks, has generally been controlled by physicians. In the United States virtually no regulation surrounds the area; physical examination, medical histories, and genetic screening of donors are not required and are thus performed haphazardly depending upon the preference of particular physicians. Nor are decisions as to appropriate sperm recipients subject to official sanctions. Physicians may select any criteria they wish in determining suitable candidates for AID motherhood and in matching donors to these recipients. From the sparse data available, it appears that values about families and masculine authority may loom large in these decisions, as might the profit motive, an issue of some consequence for a procedure which may cost as much as £66 per single insemination and when numerous inseminations may be required to effect impregnation (Curie-Cohen, Luttrell and Shapiro, 1979). Many doctors refuse outright to inseminate unmarried women, although a recent study revealed that about 9.5% of doctors responding to a questionnaire had inseminated some single women. The screening criteria which might be applied to accepting such women for insemination were not specified (Curie-Cohen, Luttrell and Shapiro, 1979).

At the same time that some women had begun to use self-help gynaecology to gain a more intimate understanding of their reproductive cycles and thus to avoid unwanted pregnancies, other women began to apply their concern with reproductive autonomy to their desire to bear children and to become mothers. Artificial insemination is simple to perform if a donor is available. If it is carried out within two hours of ejaculation, no special storage problems arise. More important for women's autonomy, however, is the fact that no special equipment or elaborate technology is needed to effect insemination. Simple household implements (such as syringes and the legendary turkey basters) may be used to deposit the sperm and the recipient's home may be the most relaxed setting for insemination.

There is nothing new, of course, about intentional single motherhood; the possibility of using a liaison with a man, whether long or short term, to launch a desired pregnancy has always been an option for single women, although the stigma attached to this choice has generally been severe. As more liberal perspectives on illegitimacy seem to have proliferated, however, and as women's involvement in the work force has increased their economic autonomy, the notion that single motherhood might occur through other than disastrous circumstances has begun to receive more general recognition.

For married women and women in relatively stable heterosexual unions, the decision to have or not to have a child may be implemented in a fairly straightforward manner. For women who lack a male partner, however, women who make up the formal category of 'single', the issue is far more complex. The ticking away of the biological clock (cf. Fabe and Wikler, 1979) and the sometimes intense desire to experience pregnancy, childbirth and motherhood must be considered in light of the massive economic problems which typically accompany single motherhood, the questions of supplying a masculine influence for a growing child, the possibly hostile responses of family, friends and community, not to mention the more basic problem of enlisting the co-operation of a suitable biological father. For lesbian women, these difficulties can be even more discouraging. Liaisons with men, however transitory, may be contemplated with distaste, and fears that a father might be able to interfere with the family or even win custody of the child later on are particularly serious considerations.

Further, some lesbians assume that doctors would be even more unwilling to inseminate them than other 'single' women and thus may anticipate difficulties trying to use established AID channels. Non-biological motherhood, adoption, appears to be an even more illusory goal, however, as the number of available children dwindles. Some adoption agencies refuse to consider applications by homosexuals; others are unwilling to place children with single parents as long as preferred two-parent homes can be found. Thus, many single women, whether or not they are lesbians, are discouraged from attempting parenthood through adoption by the lengthy investigations, the long waiting periods, the likelihood that they must adopt children who are 'difficult to place' (i.e. older, mentally or physically disabled, racially mixed), the expense, and the possibility that their investment of time, money and hope may not, with any certainty, bring them a child.

There are many lesbian women who manage to traverse these obstacles successfully and who do, in fact, become mothers by some method. Some succeed at adopting; others enter into sexual liaisons with men and conceive through what might be considered 'ordinary' means. Still others, whose motherhood may precede their lesbianism, have children from past marriages or heterosexual unions and thus closely resemble the majority of single mothers who gain that status through marital dissolution.

Still other lesbians choose to become mothers by means of artificial insemination (some prefer to call this method 'donor insemination' or more simply 'insemination'). The four cases to be discussed here represent four different approaches to AID. (While fairly representative of women interviewed in my research, these four cases represent styles of action within the AID mode, and cannot be said to be typical of any wider population.) Two of the women used medical practitioners to obtain sperm and to be impregnated; two were inseminated outside the medical establishment, taking advantage of the simplicity of AID technology. These cases illustrate ways in which the medical establishment can be circumvented, and also show that while AID can permit women to carry out conception without masculine intrusion, there is no existing method of AID which can simultaneously satisfy women's needs for both anonymity and autonomy; potential mothers selecting a pathway to pregnancy must 'make do' with limited alternatives. It appears, in addition, from these cases, that male participation in the business of becoming pregnant is not avoided merely out of feminist orthodoxy, but because it is seen to represent a threat to the future of the family in that lesbian mothers are particularly vulnerable to custody challenge (Hunter and Polikoff, 1976; Lewin, 1981).

While artificial insemination may appear to be a clear alternative to conception through sexual intercourse, it can, in fact, be brought about in a number of ways, each of which places somewhat different demands on the mother and requires different kinds of cooperation by other people, including health professionals. In selecting an approach to AID, prospective mothers who are lesbian must balance a number of considerations: their ability or desire to enlist the aid of health professionals (expense may be a key issue here), their desire to effect impregnation independently, concerns with anonymity vis-à-vis the donor, and availability of donors and/or intermediaries from their own social networks.

Joan, the mother of a four year old son, had always wanted to have a child. She was one of four children of wealthy parents and comments: 'I was really into a home–family situation . . . I wanted that nucleus, that core of a family situation'. The support provided by a private income made it unnecessary for her to work, and though she was well into her thirties she had not settled down in an occupation. In selecting to conceive by AID, she said:

> I didn't want to adopt, I wanted to have my own child. I didn't want to . . . have to sleep with a man to get him. So artificial insemination was the only way.

Arranging for AID turned out to be relatively simple. Joan approached a private doctor, who agreed to arrange insemination for her after questioning her about her financial status. She concerned herself very little with the individual characteristics of the donor, being confident that the 'donor system' took care of eliminating donors with 'hereditary diseases'. Further, she said, 'they (the donors) are all doctors, so they have to have some smarts'. In commenting on the importance of anonymity in the process, on wanting to avoid involving a man, 'some man on the street', in any way, she said: 'I wanted the total responsibility of the child . . . I guess I didn't want to take a chance of anybody trying to take him away from me'.

Another informant, the mother of a two year old daughter, had some similar concerns in choosing artificial insemination. Marilyn came from a large, conservative Catholic family, and says that she always wanted to have a baby, that children were very important in her family. When she became a lesbian during her college years, she gave the question of motherhood little thought, except to assume that she would no longer be able to achieve this valued goal. Through volunteer work with a women's health project, she learned of the existence of AID and this rekindled her interest in motherhood. She began calling various places that might supply information, concentrating on alternative health resources. A local holistic clinic, which did not specialise in AID, but whose staff had acted as intermediaries for several women, finally came to her attention, and she carried out the insemination through their facilities. Once her decision had been made, she began to plan when to perform the insemination, based on her work schedule, her insurance coverage, and a rather vague notion of when her fertile period would occur. Although she was using a health facility, she saw herself as very much in charge of the procedure. The intermediary, in her view, brought the sperm to her, 'so it was just up to me, whenever I wanted to have it done'. She made a number of specific requests about the donor's appearance and health. Once she decided on the time, and assured herself that she was ovulating, she went to the clinic and as she explained, inseminated herself, becoming pregnant on the first attempt. She had a home birth, consciously choosing to exclude attendants 'involved in the established medical system'. Although she was resolved at the time of the insemination that she never know the identity of the donor, she says that she later came to regret that she did not have 'the name of the father' put on file so that her daughter could later inquire about her origins. Interestingly, she feels strongly about entering 'unknown' under 'name of father' on the birth certificate and chose instead to draw a line through the box. 'Writing "unknown"', she said, 'sounds to me like you accidentally got pregnant or you don't know who the father is and I don't exactly know who the father is, but I do know how it came to be that I got pregnant.'

Grace, a musician in her early thirties, always assumed that she would have children at some time in her life. However, she experienced some conflicts as she developed a commitment to a career and felt unwilling to 'give up everything, which is what I felt it would have to be' in order to have a child. Thus, not until after she had become a lesbian and come to know women who were raising children without men, did she ever really consider having a child on her own: 'I had never met an unwed mother which is what we called those pitiful poor women who had children out of wedlock'. During her first years as a lesbian, however, she lived with a partner who was a mother, and became involved directly in the care of her children. This experience made her consider motherhood more seriously. She found a male friend who agreed to act as an intermediary between herself and an anonymous donor. She was quite specific about the kind of donor she wanted, with respect to race, physical appearance, and particular health conditions which might be hereditary. After many insemination efforts, she became pregnant and had a daughter. Anonymity was a priority because of her acute awareness of the problems lesbian mothers can face with child custody. Because she is active in feminist politics and is open about her lesbianism, she feels that she and her child might be particularly vulnerable to this sort of threat. On the other hand, she feels that she ought to have set up some way for her daughter to be able to eventually locate 'her biological father'. Nevertheless, she has made no concrete efforts to arrange this, fearing if she asks more of the donor than was originally agreed to, he might also ask more of her, specifically in the area of custody.

Finally, Louise, a counter-culture[1] lesbian in her early twenties who says that she always wanted to have a child, had tried unsuccessfully to become pregnant durıng past encounters with men. Until she met a woman who had had a baby through AID, she believed that as a lesbian she would never be able to have a child of her own. Once she learned about AID and determined that it was not difficult to perform, she resolved to impregnate herself. She approached several gay men she knew and asked them if they would donate sperm; after several firm rejections, she found a man who was 'thrilled' to be asked and obtained the necessary sample from him. She carried out the insemination alone in her room, with candle light and soft music, envisioning the insemination as 'a perfect baby spirit' entering her. Louise believes that she knew almost immediately that the insemination had taken. Although her delivery involved multiple interventions and was extremely traumatic physically, she also describes the birth of her daughter in mystical terms:

> It was about the best thing I ever experienced. I was totally amazed. The labour was like I had died . . . I had just died. The

minute she came out, I was born again. It was like we'd just been born together.

The birth led to a number of important changes in her life: a temporary reconciliation with her mother, and a great deal of supportive interaction with her father, with whom she had not been on the best of terms. She feels that motherhood has influenced her to regularise her life in terms of relationships ('I choose my friends very carefully'), an emphasis on being responsible and alert ('I don't get drunk anymore'), and a growing concern with cleanliness and order. Although she was acquainted with the biological father, and he was aware that she had become pregnant, she is careful to avoid any further contact with him. She moved to another city after becoming pregnant. She knows only his first name and was careful that he did not know her name, or whereabouts. While she feels that it would be desirable for her daughter to meet her father, she says: 'I just don't trust him. I feel really threatened in general about child custody things. A little bit, by my being a lesbian I feel like it's a threat; my being poor is a threat'. Because of her fears about challenges to her custody, she not only avoids her daughter's biological father but hopes that her appearance and demeanour enable her to blend into the general population, not to stand out as a lesbian. 'It's like this deep down fear that someone might really like her and decide that her mother is a lesbian and therefore, she's unfit . . . They will never get my child, but they might try.'

These four cases present a continuum of reproductive decision making used by lesbian women. They range from Joan's reliance on her doctor to do everything, through Marilyn's use of a facility on her own terms, to Grace's avoidance of a medical setting but her use of an intermediary, and finally Louise's autonomous self-insemination. On another level, these variations with respect to the use of medical services also represent variations in the maintenance of anonymity. At one extreme, Joan left the selection of the donor up to her doctor, and not only doesn't know his name, but has no personal specifications which might supply him with a shadowy identity. At the other end of the continuum, Louise, though concerned about anonymity, has met her donor and knows his first name. Marilyn and Grace fall roughly in the middle. Both made particular characteristics paramount in requesting donors, and thus know at least that much about their children's biological fathers. Marilyn's donor was obtained through an impersonal agency, which solidifies his anonymity, while Grace relied upon an extension of her friendship network, which has greater potential for compromising anonymity. In three of the cases, the need to maintain anonymity is strongly emphasised and in all of these cases the fear of loss of custody looms large in reinforcing this concern. Standing somewhat in conflict with the maintenance of anonymity, however, is the concern three of the mothers voiced with providing a means for their children to locate their fathers at some later date, though none of them has found a way to meet this need without seriously undermining anonymity.

The variations which appear in these four cases indicate the ways in which AID can leave room for women to achieve varying levels of autonomy in becoming mothers. The absence of biological fathers alone does not insure that insemination and birth will be experienced as self-determined acts. Joan, for example, had a male doctor perform the insemination; her concern was more directed to the outcome (her own baby) than to her own autonomy during the process. Her insistence on excluding the biological father was based less on ideology than on anxiety about her status as a lesbian mother. In contrast, for Louise, the insemination and birth were intensely personal, even mystical, experiences, and she emphasised her nearly total control of the insemination. While she finally had a highly medicalised delivery, she dwells very little on this in describing her experience; rather, she views her daughter and herself as beginning a new life together, one in which she can make conscious decisions and choices and over which the rest of the world has little control. For all the women discussed here, autonomy resides more in the ability to manipulate varying levels of self-determination and anonymity, than in an ideological commitment to separatism or a denial of the masculine element in reproduction.

Conclusion

The study of women has allowed many disciplines, anthropology among them, to move into new areas of enquiry, resulting in the broadening of our understanding of the varieties of female experience and the meaning of gender categories. In many cases, this new interest has brought a clearer comprehension of matters which have wider relevance in the general discipline. Such is the case, for example, in anthropology, where the study of women led us to investigate more thoroughly the informal domains of human societies. Similarly, our interest in motherhood has intensified in the context of our new sub-field. Nevertheless, this expanded interest and the wealth of new data it has supplied have, for the most part, implicitly rested on a belief that motherhood is a basic condition to which women must adapt and that the character of that adaptation will determine other features of women's participation in society and culture.

In contrast, I have suggested we view women as rational beings, as strategists, who use motherhood as a resource within the context of on-going strategies. As a dynamic dimension of these strategies motherhood is both something one uses to adapt to existing conditions as well as a condition to which one must adapt. This model is not unlike the more transactional, interactive approaches which have been proposed in recent years for the study of social organisation and which have been applied to such areas as ethnicity with extremely productive results (cf. Barth, 1969). Just as Barth and others have suggested that the apparently 'given' category of ethnicity can be manipulated and used strategically, thus enriching our whole approach to social organisation, it seems to me that breaking apart motherhood can bring us closer to a more dynamic appreciation of women's cultural and social behaviour.

Abandonment of a monolithic concept of motherhood presents a further advantage to the cultural anthropologist. Like other cultural domains, such as kinship and religion, motherhood may be understood analytically to stand as a microcosm of the wider culture; that is, close examination of its various features reveals the structures, values, and contradictions which characterise the society in which it is embedded. The centrality of the individual and the related emphasis on the full realisation of the self which are stressed in the American version of intentional single motherhood exemplify this sort of application.

The issue of women's strategies becomes particularly vital when one attempts an understanding of behaviour in medical settings and the way in which women use health care services. Women are not only primary consumers of health care (by virtue of paying more visits to doctors), but are the mediators and negotiators who interpret the sickness behaviour of those close to them and decide whether or not to direct them to health care providers (Graham, 1984a). In the course of becoming mothers, they are also likely to interact intensively with the health care system and, even under conditions of physician dominance, to make a variety of decisions about care options, diet, exercise, and providers. As the range of choices presented by the obstetrical world continues to expand, both because of response to consumer demands (Ruzek, 1980) and because of the proliferation of high technology interventions (for example, amniocentesis, ultra-sound diagnosis, foetal heart monitors) women's motivations and goals will have an ever-increasing significance in shaping their birth experiences. This may prove to be especially important as the incidence of so-called delayed childbearing rises and the numbers of over-35 first time mothers (called 'elderly primiparas' in medical terminology) soar. These women are likely to be highly purposeful in their entry into motherhood at the same time that they are candidates *par excellence* for obstetrical intervention of every description. The conflicts they encounter in medical settings and the resolutions reached will be difficult to understand without an awareness of the varying goals women pursue through motherhood. Thus, the strategic approach proposed here does more I think, than introduce new terminological complications and other disciplinary conceits; it points to a dimension needed in basic research on women if it is to be usefully applied to the solution of real problems.

Note

1. The term 'counter-culture' was popularised by Theodore Roszak (1969) in his study of the rebellious youth culture of the 1960s. Members of this 'culture' were identified as rebelling against middle class values particularly by rejecting consumerism, conventional sexual morality, regular employment, and hierarchical education and by embracing mystical (usually Eastern) religious experience and the use of psychedelic drugs.

Acknowledgements

The research reported here was supported by a grant from the National Institute of Mental Health, #30890. I would like to acknowledge the invaluable assistance of Terrie A. Lyons who worked on the project throughout the planning and data collection phases and conducted some of the preliminary analyses. I also received able clerical assistance from Beverly Cubbage and Andrea Temkin. A number of colleagues have commented on various versions of this study and have helped me to clarify my ideas. I would like to thank, in particular, Carole Browner, Louisa Flander, Carol Shepherd McClain, Virginia Olesen and Sheryl Ruzek for their suggestions. The incisive comments of Ann W. Merrill throughout the preparation of this work have been especially important to me, as have been her patience and support. Earlier versions of this chapter were presented at the meetings of the Society for Applied Anthropology, Edinburgh, Scotland (1981) and at Cornell and Stanford Universities (1983).

9 Discomforts in Pregnancy: Traditional Remedies and Medical Prescriptions

Hilary Homans

Women receive conflicting images of what it means to be pregnant. The most extreme images we are presented with are either that pregnancy is women's most 'natural' condition, something we should all aspire towards, or the clinical view which stresses the pathological aspects of pregnancy and medical intervention in the management of pregnancy. These images obviously contradict each other, while at the same time do not match the reality of women's experiences. When we look more closely at the image of pregnancy as women's destiny, we find that it really only applies to white, middle class married women of certain ages and parity (see Graham, 1977a), and women who fall into these categories have themselves written about the tensions they experienced in becoming mothers (Rich, 1977b; Weare, 1979). On the other hand, the clinical view is manifested in the relatively isolated hospital or general practitioner antenatal visits, although these encounters may be extremely distressing and the effect of them very pervasive (Haire, 1972; Stoller Shaw, 1974; Oakley, 1975).

Many women do not live up to the image of being in tune with nature (blossoming, blooming and radiant are words often used to describe pregnant women), nor do they see themselves suffering from a potentially pathological condition. Rather their health tends to fluctuate on a daily basis and they are almost certain to suffer from some discomforts (such as digestive disorders, aches and pains).

> I am fit now, but I don't know about tomorrow. (Manjit, first pregnancy)

> I'm better now. I felt sick and had pains in me stomach early on. (Sandra, fourth pregnancy)

These discomforts (particularly nausea and vomiting) have been described by a variety of writers as psychogenic in origin and as a reaction *against* pregnancy (Deutsch, 1944; de Beauvoir, 1972). This is despite the fact that there is no scientific evidence for such an assertion (Lennane and Lennane, 1973, p. 289).

Medical texts say that morning sickness is 'always more marked in neurotic subjects' (Davies *et al.* 1939, p. 64) and 'may indicate resentment, ambivalence and inadequacy in women ill-prepared for motherhood' (Benson, 1972). This presumably means that those women who are not totally committed to fulfilling their femininity by becoming a mother will express their reaction through sickness.

A consequence of this line of thought for pregnant women is that their symptoms are not taken seriously. As Lennane and Lennane say: 'There is unfortunately a widespread view that the patient whose symptoms are psychogenic is not entitled to any symptomatic relief' (1973, p. 291). Also, the very commonness of nausea and vomiting and the fact that the majority of pregnant women suffer such symptoms may mean that doctors perceive them as a 'normal' state in pregnancy. Or as Zola (1979) says as 'natural and inevitable and thus to be ignored as of no consequence' (p. 44).

Given the high incidence of discomforts in pregnancy it is worthwhile to ask whether women themselves perceive these to be a problem, and if so how they cope with them. This chapter therefore addresses women's perceptions of health and illness in pregnancy and the sources of advice and information women draw on to alleviate suffering caused by discomforts. It appears that in the first instance many women will draw on their own knowledge, or that of older women and female friends, and use home remedies to deal with discomforts. Women who do not have ready access to such sources of knowledge may either consult a local chemist or their general practitioner. The contradictory way in which some members of the medical profession view discomforts in pregnancy tends to determine the treatment women receive.

The data for this chapter comes from seventy-eight women who were interviewed at their first visit to a consultant antenatal clinic in a midlands city. Fifty-two of these women were interviewed again in their own homes at eight months pregnant when they spoke at length about their health and illness during pregnancy and their use of the maternal health services. Half of the women in each of these samples are white British women and half are British women of Asian origin. The majority of the latter group had migrated from the Punjab in India[1] and for the purpose of this chapter will be referred to as Punjabi women. In many ways the strategies the women use in dealing with discomforts are similar and have their own internal logic relating to folk beliefs about health and illness, or they are a pragmatic response to what sources of information are available and accessible.

There is now considerable literature referring to the particular problems that black and ethnic minority groups experience in obtaining health care which is appropriate to their needs (Mitchell and Wilson,

1981; Satow and Homans, 1981; Homans and Satow, 1982; Donovan, 1983; Torkington, 1983). This literature represents a conscious attempt to challenge earlier writings about black and ethnic minority groups which see 'them' as a 'problem' or 'different'. For instance, previous studies have looked at the way Asian mothers differ from white mothers in terms of being 'older, shorter, and almost always married' with 'poorer nutritional status' (Smalley and Bissenden, 1977, p. 408) and the 'demand' they make on the health services is assessed without in any way measuring their health 'needs' (Ronalds *et al.* 1977, p. 283). The way in which Asian women have been presented in research studies has been comprehensively criticised (Parmar, 1982). Whether these problems can be avoided by a white author, however aware of the issues, is a moot point. The challenge that black and ethnic minorities now face is one of drawing together their own research and literature and re-writing their history (Carby, 1982), a process already under way (e.g. Wilson, 1978).

Perceptions of health and illness during pregnancy

Health is often assumed to be a constant state. A person is either 'healthy' or 'ill' and to be 'ill' usually implies having the condition legitimated by a medically qualified person (Parsons, 1951). But looking at health and illness in this way fails to account for most people's experiences, particularly in relation to minor ailments, for example, coughs, colds and discomforts of pregnancy. In these instances most of us continue as 'normal' and use self medication, either home cures or chemical compounds purchased at the chemist. A study of the incidence of symptoms (Dunnell and Cartwright, 1972) found that although 83 per cent of the sample rated their health as good or excellent during a two week period, 91 per cent of them had experienced some symptoms. It therefore seems that illness is 'a feature of everyday life' (Herxheimer and Stimson, 1981, p. 48).

During pregnancy, women generally perceive themselves to be healthy, although they also suffer from discomforts. Of the women studied 76 per cent described their health in positive terms at their first interview (see Table 1).

The dynamic nature of pregnancy, however, and the continual fluctuations in health in pregnancy leads us to question the usefulness of analysing pregnancy in terms of the adoption of the sick role as some writers in the functionalist tradition do (for example, Hern, 1971, 1975; Rosengren, 1961–62; Goshen-Gottstein, 1966). For the state of health of the woman in pregnancy can often be related to her non-pregnant perception of health, and this is a factor which has been excluded from writings to date on the adoption of the sick role in pregnancy. It is important to relate changes in health at this time to the

Table 1 Women's Description of their State of Health during Pregnancy

Initial sample N = 78		Total No.	Total %
Positive responses	Same as usual	6	8
	Good/Fine	16	20
	All right	26	33
	Very good/Very well	11	14
Negative responses	Poor	7	9
	Not very well	3	4
	Rotten/Terrible	3	4
	Suicidal	1	1
	Bit depressed	2	3
	Better now	3	4
	Total	78	100
	Positive responses	59	76
	Negative responses	19	24
		78	100

woman's non-pregnant state of health, for although women do experience discomforts during pregnancy, some women even feel healthier.

> I've been marvellous all the way through, I've just got fatter and that's it. I'm the same as I am when I'm normal. I don't even get tired, you know, people say you'll get ever so tired, but in fact I think I've got more energy. 'Cos I can't sleep at night, you see, 'cos you can't get comfortable. So I'm up earlier in the mornings now and doing my washing and God knows what. (Annette, first pregnancy)

Although three quarters of the women described their health in positive terms, this is not to say they felt well throughout their pregnancy. The women were at different stages of pregnancy and the complaints they suffered from varied: pains in the stomach, digestive disorders, tiredness, giddiness, backache, feeling lazy, and trouble with walking. When they were interviewed again at eight months pregnant they recounted the discomforts they had suffered from. *All* of the women reported experiencing at least one discomfort and 88 per cent said they had suffered from more than one complaint. The main discomforts for the white women were – heartburn 61.5 per cent; sickness 58 per cent; aches and pains 35 per cent and indigestion 31 per cent. The Punjabi women suffered most from weakness or tiredness 77 per cent; vomiting 58 per cent; heartburn 15 per cent and difficulty in moving 15 per cent. For *all* women the most common discomfort was vomiting or sickness, 58 per cent of all the women suffered with this; followed by weakness or tiredness 44 per cent; and heartburn 38 per cent. None of the women spontaneously mentioned such 'secret complaints' as vaginal discharge and cystitis referred to by Graham in her study (1977b).

Women's perception of discomforts during pregnancy varied according to their own experience of pregnancy. All the first-time pregnant women of course had no previous experience of the body changes which take place in pregnancy and have no yardstick to measure these changes by. They did not know for instance whether the discomforts were indications of something wrong in the pregnancy, and a few first-time pregnant women did not automatically associate the discomfort with the fact of being pregnant. This was particularly the case with those women who did not know they were pregnant.

> I thought it was a haddock I'd had at college, it was horrible and I was being sick after it, and I blamed it [the sickness] on that. I had it for a few weeks, but I only started having it after the haddock.
> HH: Did you know that you were pregnant then?
> Well I thought I might have been, but I thought it [the sickness] was the haddock and it put me off fried foods as well. (Tessa, first pregnancy)

> My mother told me when I was pregnant. When I started vomiting – I didn't know – then my mother told me. (Zorda, speaking of her first pregnancy)

Women who had been pregnant before and therefore knew what to expect during pregnancy often compared the discomforts they experienced in each of their pregnancies. Differences between the pregnancies were often accounted for in terms of changes in social circumstances.

> I was at work before as well [in previous pregnancy] you see, right up to eight months, and that made a lot of difference, 'cos you're with people all the time, with girls, like. And you're not

> sitting thinking about how poorly you feel or how tired you feel . . . Once I'm on my feet and working I'm alright, it's when I'm sitting down I start and feel tired and heavy and not much energy. (Lorraine, second pregnancy)

Women with young children often cited the children as the reason for their tiredness in this pregnancy.

> My husband often says to me 'Why don't you have a rest in the afternoon' . . . But what am I supposed to do with her? . . . I can't handle her . . . I'm tired, I could quite happily go to sleep . . . but I can't 'cos she's always there. Sometimes I'm so tired, I'm so worn out. (Janet, second pregnancy)

> I do feel more tired [in this pregnancy] – well, from six o'clock in the morning he's [eighteen month old son] like a little dynamo you see . . . He's on the go all the time. (Mary, second pregnancy)

Other changes in social circumstances were seen as the cause of women's poor health, for instance, one woman's husband left her when she was three months' pregnant and another one's mother died:

> I do not keep well these days. I feel very weak. In the previous pregnancies I never felt like this. This time I am not feeling well at all . . . At first I felt quite well, but now I have started getting very weak. It's since my mother died. (Kashmir, fifth pregnancy)

The woman whose husband had left her recorded the largest number of complaints, suggesting a relationship between stress and ill health:

> I've had morning sickness, heartburn, strain pains, (and that was before the baby turned!) varicose veins, aches, pains, swelling . . . I'm beginning to think I'm becoming a hypochondriac. (Maureen, first pregnancy)

There are thus social factors which affect a woman's state of health when she is pregnant and it is important to recognise the presence of these social factors when attempting to understand how women perceive their health in pregnancy.

Social factors are also important in determining the women's tolerance of the discomfort she experiences. For instance, a woman who is in paid employment outside the home may find it difficult to continue her job while suffering from morning sickness. As one woman said:

> I was very sick with Carol . . . well actually, I was a bit cowardly actually 'cos as I say I was working at the time and I was having

> to leave classes and be sick. Yeah, every day I was having it – it was alright if you like, but it was getting a bit embarrassing. (Ann – teacher)

In this case, the woman found the sickness was preventing her from teaching (and was causing her embarrassment), so she sought relief from the discomfort which she said she would have tolerated under other circumstances. We will now turn to the measures women took to maintain or restore health during pregnancy.

Health maintenance

One of the main determinants of whether a woman sought relief for pregnancy discomforts was if she felt it was possible to control the condition, or whether it was 'all part of pregnancy'. In the same way that women's perceptions of discomforts varied depending on whether or not they had been pregnant before, so did their knowledge of maintaining health, even though most women had relatives and friends willing to give advice and they all received a copy of the English language publication *You and your baby* from the hospital clinic.[2]

Maintaining health during pregnancy was seen as important by all the women studied and 81 per cent of the sample could name specific things which would help them remain healthy. The majority of Punjabi women (72 per cent) placed importance on diet, while the white women were more likely to mention exercise (41 per cent) and fresh air as their prescription for maintaining health during pregnancy.

The Punjabi women's stress on diet for maintaining health is consistent with traditional Indian medical knowledge which considers a 'faulty' diet to be the main cause of illness. Within India the traditional Hindu system of medicine (Ayurveda), places emphasis on maintaining a balance, or equilibrium, in the body by paying attention to the amount of 'hot' and 'cold' foods eaten. During illness, balance can be restored by adjusting the amount of 'hot' or 'cold' food eaten (Homans, 1983, pp. 74–5). According to Ayurveda, pregnancy is a time when changes are taking place in women's bodies, and these changes need to be balanced by alterations in diet (Nichter, 1977, p. 94). For the women studied there was a marked prohibition of 'hot' foods in early pregnancy, when the foetus is seen to be most vulnerable. The women learnt about these prohibitions from older Punjabi women, either in India or in Britain, and they formed part of a very co-ordinated belief system about the importance of diet in maintaining health (Homans, 1983).

Knowledge about the importance of diet in health maintenance was much more fragmented for the white women, although also based on the concept of balance. They referred to a 'well balanced diet' according to Western nutritional science, and the avoidance of foods which did not 'agree' with them (cf. Homans, 1983). The working class white women were like the Punjabi women in that they learnt about food prohibitions during pregnancy from older women (usually their mother or mother-in-law). These older women also have knowledge of traditional ways of coping with the discomforts of pregnancy. Home cures, or the appropriate course of action to take, are part of what traditionally constitutes women's knowledge, sometimes derogatorily referred to as 'old wives' tales' (Chamberlain, 1981). Female knowledge of healing dates back centuries when wise women were respected for their skills in treating everyday maladies (Ehrenreich and English, 1978). This knowledge has been passed down by generations of experienced women and in rural India it is still the older women of the household who have knowledge of *desi* (home cures). In Britain there is a much more fragmented body of knowledge about traditional remedies for certain maladies, and in many cases this knowledge has been undermined by western curative medicine (i.e. allopathy).

Health restoration

Traditional recipes or folk medicine

There is a substantial body of literature which suggests that folk medicines and traditional remedies are mainly used in countries which do not have a co-ordinated system of allopathic medicine. Within this literature there are several assumptions: (1) folk treatments are associated with 'poverty and ignorance' (Blum and Kreitman, 1983, p. 123); (2) that allopathic medicine is superior to other forms of traditional medicine and the population needs to become 'acculturated' so that western medicine gains 'primacy in the hierarchy of resort' (Schwartz, 1969, p. 208); and finally, it is assumed that folk medicine is only used in strange, exotic cultures and does not exist in the western world.

Yet there is evidence to suggest that people in Britain rely on traditional remedies, or folk medicines, for minor illnesses and that most illnesses are contained within the community with some form of self-medication, including home remedies (Herxheimer and Stimson, 1981, pp. 56–7; Dunnell and Cartwright, 1972). It is also interesting to note that in the 'western' world there is currently a revival of interest in folk remedies and their curative properties, particularly in relation to women's health (Beckett, 1973; Seaman and Seaman, 1978; Phillips and Rakusen, 1979; Chamberlain, 1981; and Reitz, 1981).

In the sample studied, the Punjabi women were more likely to have knowledge of traditional recipes for the discomforts of pregnancy (73 per cent), compared with the white women (35 per cent). For digestive disorders, changes in diet were universally prescribed, while for other discomforts, such as tiredness and giddiness, a certain course of action was advised. Although the Punjabi women were more knowledgeable about traditional recipes than the white women, there are similarities in some of the recipes used.

In the case of vomiting and sickness the Punjabi women were likely to avoid 'hot' foods, while the white women mentioned recipes they used for coping with the sickness:

> I'm not eating 'hot' things . . . chillies and peppers my mother told me not to eat. (Kiran)

> I had bicarbonate of soda – I mean everybody takes that. (Margaret)

> I do my home cures. For sickness, I've got a basic thing I've used for years. I make it myself – it's a kind of soup with pasta, it's very thin and salty. And I drink chamomile tea and things like that, it has a sort of settling effect. (Barbara)

For heartburn the traditional remedy also lies in an alteration of diet. Both Punjabi and white women mentioned drinking milk as the cure for heartburn, though the reasons they gave for the ameliorative affect of milk on heartburn, came out of two completely different philosophies. Punjabi women saw the prescription of a 'cooling' food such as milk to be essential in restoring the proper balance in the body and thereby reducing the burning sensation.

> Two months ago I had quite a lot of heartburn, and my mother told me to put some glucose in milk and drink it at night. It does help, especially at night if I have it before I go to sleep. It stops the burning. (Jaswinder)

British women on the other hand, consider milk to be important in restoring the acid/alkali balance in the stomach:

> I drink the top of the milk – if you have it before you eat something, it stops you getting it [heartburn]. Just take a teaspoon of cream . . . it stops you making too much acid in your stomach. It does work. (Janice)

Both groups of women saw fried foods as causing the heartburn and they would try and avoid these foods. The white women mentioned eating late at night as another cause of heartburn, and would remedy this by eating earlier:

> You occasionally get heartburn if you eat too much late at night . . . I remedied it by not eating anything after tea-time . . . It was something I could control myself. (Rachel)

> Funnily enough she'd [mother] been saying today with this heartburn, she'd been telling me one or two bits of pieces to keep off . . . She said avoid pastry um . . . a lot of fat foods, anything that's too fatty, like you know. (Caroline)

They also mentioned taking bicarbonate of soda, lemonade and Polo mints to relieve the heartburn:

> With the third one I had bad heartburn and I ate packets and packets of Polo mints . . . My aunty was a nurse and when she was pregnant she used to have medicine from the doctor and there was mint in it. So I'll have that. (Sandra)

Indigestion was also seen to be caused by eating the wrong foods, or eating at the 'wrong time' of day. The prescription for indigestion therefore involved a change in diet:

> I'd had some fish and chips the other Monday from the chip shop and I really enjoyed it at the time. But all evening I felt I was in labour almost . . . It's as if I've got to stick rigidly to an earlier time. (Diane)

The other digestive disorder women suffered from during pregnancy was constipation. This condition was often aggravated by the taking of iron tablets and some of the women did not take the iron tablets because of this. However, most of the women would alter their diet in an attempt to alleviate the discomfort. The Punjabi women had several traditional recipes they used as a cure for constipation, while the white women ate more roughage.

> I've eaten a lot of vegetables and tried to eat more fruit and all things like that . . . I've taken a cereal in the morning which I really detest . . . I must try and keep myself regular. And having iron tablets, well, I don't normally have any problems like that. But I decided myself to take bran and Alpen, which I hate, but I push it down. (Ann)

> For constipation I will take *banaksha* only. [A herbal tea containing eucalyptus] (Surinder)

> For constipation you can take sweet *saunf* [aniseed] or *pahardi saunf* [mountain aniseed] or put *juan* [barley] or the petals of rose flowers, or *banaksha* [herbal tea containing eucalyptus] – things like this, which are made into a *kahra* which is like tea. You can boil all these in milk and drink that. (Rajinder)

In addition to these traditional recipes, the women had different social definitions of illness and corresponding cures. For instance, Punjabi women referred to cures for 'bad blood', 'weakness', aches and pains, 'breathing trouble' and high blood pressure. 'Bad blood' or 'bloodlessness', is a recognised illness according to Ayurveda and is caused by certain foodstuffs. Milk, for instance, is thought to raise the quality of the blood. When a woman is pregnant she is more likely to suffer from 'bad blood' or 'bloodlessness' and feel weak:

> My mother said 'Your blood might be bad you know' for these itchings like [the woman had come out in a rash during her pregnancy] so she said 'eat some honey like'. (Gurbax)

> I feel very weak. Just look how dark and pale I look. I feel weak and breathless and I can't sit down comfortably and I can't walk, my legs feel weak and shaky. When I get up after a sleep I feel I'm going to fall down – when the 'heat' rises in me I feel faint and fall down. (Gurmej)

The Indian remedy for weakness and 'bloodlessness' is eating strengthening foods such as almonds (see Homans, 1983, p. 78).

> The people at home tell me to have almonds and butter for my health and to stop the weakness. (Ramesh)

The white women also suffered from weakness and 'bloodlessness' and had traditional methods of coping with these complaints which did not involve a change in diet:

> I seem to get giddy turns if I'm not careful. And I know I'm going a bit pale in my face, or perhaps I've been on my feet too long. I know I've got to sit down . . . Well I had it four or five times with Rebecca but I was always able to control it, because I always knew it was coming on, so I knew I had to sit down, just till it blowed over, just a few minutes. (Janet)

Other recipes the Punjabi women mentioned as cures for discomforts in pregnancy were:

> When my back aches, I have *sundh* [dry ginger] in butter and with sugar. (Surinder)

> Yesterday she [mother-in-law] was after me, because I said 'I've got a pain in my back'. And she said 'You've got to have almonds oil'. (Kiran)

> When I had the third baby I had some breathing trouble and I used to take the Indian treatment of having *saunf* [aniseed] and only then could I breathe at night. (Charanjit)

> Take cloves for blood pressure, with honey. Take a spoonful of honey with a clove in it – it's good for high blood pressure . . . It also purifies the blood. (Surinder)

All of the women quoted above learnt about traditional recipes for the discomforts of pregnancy from older women. The Punjabi women had either learnt the recipes in India or since they had been in Britain. As one woman said:

> In India we seldom go to the doctor. Whenever anyone is unwell the older ladies are consulted and they usually give something. (Sanjit)

Whilst the Punjabi women were twice as likely as the white women to have knowledge about traditional recipes and home cures, it appears that this knowledge is declining amongst those Punjabi women who do not have older female relatives in Britain to learn the skills from. As the quote above shows, older women are the first people consulted in the case of illness in India. With migration, families have been disrupted and for some women there is no guarantee that an older female relative is available to offer advice. Two-thirds of the Punjabi women did have relatives living in the same city compared with 92 per cent of the white women, though the Punjabi women were more likely to be living in an extended family (42 per cent) compared with the white women (12 per cent).

Another reason for the decline in use of traditional remedies by Punjabi women in Britain is the existence of the National Health Service (NHS). As medical treatment is free under the NHS, Punjabi women are able to use allopathic medicine without fear of the cost (although there may be other barriers to obtaining appropriate treatment, cf. Mitchell and Wilson, 1981). A considerable number of Punjabi women consulted their GP about discomforts in pregnancy and used medical prescriptions either on their own, or in conjunction with home cures. One Punjabi woman said she did not use *desi* (home cures) because her doctor had told her not to do so, but to take any illness to him for treatment.

The white women who used traditional recipes also consulted their GP if the discomfort persisted, or if they were worried that the discomfort indicated something was wrong. However, they also mentioned another form of self-medication, which was over-the-counter drugs available from chemists.

The chemist's shop

Manufactured drugs such as analgesics, laxatives and digestives are likely to be found in most households. Dunnell and Cartwright (1972) surveyed a sample of households in the UK and found that 99 per cent of them contained medicines of some description. On average each household had 7.3 items of non-prescribed medicines. It is possible to regard these compounds as 'the Western equivalent of medicinal herbs' (Herxheimer and Stimson, 1981, p. 51).

In the present study, it was only the white women who mentioned buying over-the-counter drugs for the discomforts of pregnancy, although another study (Donovan, 1983) shows that Asian households do contain these drugs. Forty-six per cent of the white women bought drugs for heartburn, indigestion, aches and pains. Half of the white women suffering from heartburn obtained some form of relief from the chemist's; the other women obtained relief using traditional recipes.

> I just take a little Morland or something like that. They're just indigestion, heartburn tablets – we've always got some in the house. I just take them. (Harriet)

> Once when I had it very bad I did take some, I think it was Boots make of um . . . Alka Seltzer stuff, you know. I did take some of that once because it was so bad you know. (Diane)

For indigestion the women mentioned taking Rennies or Settlers four times more often than they mentioned altering their diet to prevent the indigestion. Some women also mentioned the large amount of these tablets that they consumed.

> I'm Rennies mad! I eat a packet of twenty-four Rennies every week . . . perhaps more . . . I eat them like sweets I'm afraid. (Hazel)

> I've taken about twenty tablets in the last two days. (Maureen)

Other women were slightly more cautious of taking these tablets and only took them as a *last resort*:

> I try and *go as long* as I can actually, then I take Rennies or Settlers. I do take them, that is something I do take occasionally, but it's very rare . . . And I feel as though they are *safe* to take. (Emphasis added.) (Tessa)

It is interesting to note that some women who said they would not take drugs in pregnancy bought over-the-counter drugs. These were assumed to be safe because of their accessibility. It was often said that it was more convenient to pop down to the chemist for relief from digestive discomforts than to go to the doctor. Also some women expressed concern over the safety of prescribed drugs (as we shall see later). For some women the chemist stocked everything they needed for minor illnesses:

> There's nothing you can't get now, there's a marvellous array of stuff at the chemist. And the chemist at the Co-op Mr M. is a marvellous man, I've never known a pharmacist like him. He'll come out and explain all about the drugs to you and you can ask him about side effects and he'll get his sheet out . . . He'll tell you anything. Almost as good to tell you the truth as going to the doctor. (Janet)

The accessibility of folk remedies and over-the-counter drugs made them attractive to most of the women studied. Also they were likely to be administered by someone who was known to the women, and in the case of folk medicines particularly, this person's knowledge was likely to be trusted because they had experienced the discomforts of pregnancy themselves. Women who consulted their doctor for symptomatic relief often found themselves confronted with different views of prescribing practice and scarce practical advice.

Medical prescriptions

Medical prescriptions for discomforts were sought by those pregnant women who were unable to successfully treat the condition with home remedies or over-the-counter drugs, together with women who did not have access to this knowledge or did not consider self-medication to be efficacious. On seeking medical treatment for discomforts of pregnancy the women often became involved in a medical debate about whether or not pregnant women should be given prescribed drugs. We therefore find that some doctors refuse to prescribe drugs to pregnant women and that some women, having been given prescribed drugs, doubt their 'safety' and fail to take them. This section looks at some of the factors affecting prescribing practice and how the women studied responded to these.

It appears that within the medical profession the image of pregnancy as a potentially pathological condition is most likely to be subscribed to by obstetricians and hospital doctors (Homans, 1980, p. 496; Graham and Oakley, 1981). General practitioners (GPs), on the other hand, are more likely to be concerned with 'checking normality' (Homans, 1980, p. 496) and are often considered to be more 'interested in people' (Bruhn and Parsons, 1964; Harris, 1981). Also it has been suggested that GPs' diagnoses and treatments are couched in terms consistent with lay beliefs about health and illness (Helman, 1978). However, doctors are generally regarded as having 'special knowledge' (Freidson, 1960, p. 375) and patients usually expect them to be able to cure their illnesses.

Other factors which affect doctor–patient interaction relate to the sex, race and class of the patient. As we know, doctors are predominantly white, middle class, males (Elston, 1977; Robson *et al.* 1977; Smith, 1980; Day, 1982) and are therefore likely to have life experiences very different from those of the majority of their patients. Some of the literature relating to the problems black and ethnic minority groups experience in obtaining appropriate health care has already been discussed; other literature refers to the way that women's illnesses are often not taken seriously by male doctors (Barrett and Roberts, 1978; Doyal, 1979, pp. 215–38), the particular difficulties working class patients experience in communicating with their doctor (Cartwright, 1976), or cultural variations in communication (Homans and Satow, 1982).

In the case of the discomforts of pregnancy we find that these tensions in the doctor–patient relationship are compounded by whether or not GPs thought the condition should be relieved by prescribed medication, and we find that the GPs fall into two categories – the non-prescribers and prescribers. The first group considered that discomforts were all part of pregnancy and 'nothing to worry about' and the second group treated discomforts as they did other illnesses, i.e. they were conditions which could be alleviated with the prescription of a drug.

Non-prescribers These GPs tended to view pregnancy more as a 'natural' condition and the advice they gave closely reflected that in the clinic leaflet *You and your baby* (BMA, 1975). In the section on 'keeping well' Professor Rhodes says that morning sickness 'though unpleasant, is certainly nothing to worry about' (p. 43); breathlessness is common and 'as long as your doctor found heart and lungs normal . . . there is no need to worry' (p. 44); palpitation 'virtually only occurs in normal hearts' (p. 44); and faintness and dizziness 'are extremely common symptoms in early pregnancy' (p. 44). Similarly, an obstetric text book for nurses recognises the widespread incidence of discomforts which are 'of limited importance to the doctor or midwife, but may cause the woman herself much unhappiness and discomfort' (Garland *et al.* 1976, p. 60).

The doctors who subscribed to the view that discomforts were 'nothing to worry about' sometimes managed to allay women's anxieties about their health:

> I've just felt tired. I started getting backache and I started getting palpitations. I didn't know what they were until I asked the doctor and he explained that it was *nothing to worry about.* (Emphasis added) (Maureen – first pregnancy)

> I just can't walk. I've told him (doctor) . . . I said 'I have a bit of trouble you know getting across [the road] ' and he said 'If that's all that's wrong with you, *you haven't got nothing to worry about*'. (Emphasis added) (Sandra – fourth pregnancy)

Other women though found that this explanation did not allay their fears and they were not provided with any advice about how to alleviate the condition which to them was unique.

> It was like a blackout really. I mentioned it to the doctor, but I don't think he was all that concerned. (Janet)

> I asked the doctor what caused the rash. He said that it often happens when you're pregnant. But last time I didn't get it. When I told this to the doctor, he said 'Not all pregnancies are the same, some take 38 weeks, some take 40 . . . Sometimes you have a girl, sometimes you have a boy. It doesn't mean you have to have the same thing'. (Kiran)

Although these women were dissatisfied with the response that their ailment was all part of pregnancy, there was a further small group of women whose faith in the medical profession led them to accept the doctor's definition of their symptom as 'normal' and ceased to worry about it on the grounds that 'they would have told me if anything was wrong'. This view was also expressed in the context of negative re-assurance in consultant ante-natal clinic encounters (Homans, 1982, p. 252).

> When I stand up a lot I feel dizzy . . . I think it's because me blood doesn't flow so quickly, because I always get a lot of pins and needles in my legs and arms. They took blood tests for haemoglobin and that, so if there was anything wrong there, they would have found it, so I didn't bother saying nothing. It's got 'well' on the card 'cos I had a peep at it. (June – first pregnancy)

None of the women quoted above were given any advice about how they could alleviate the discomfort. Some women who felt a medical prescription might relieve the suffering were told that the doctor did not agree with the prescription of drugs in pregnancy.

> I told the doctor last time . . . He said 'No. You can't have any tablets while you're pregnant'. No-one had mentioned it before then. (Ramesh)

> My GP said he didn't think it was a good idea to take even Aspirin in pregnancy. (Wendy)

Only one woman out of the total sample said that her doctor had given her some advice about how to ease the condition she was suffering from and this closely resembled the traditional remedies mentioned earlier.

> I said to him [GP] that I couldn't sleep at all well, and he says 'Have a short walk and have a hot shower before you go to bed'. He said 'You have to start taking it easy now'. As I say, with him you do feel as you can ask him a little you know, whereas with the others I feel uneasy. (Sandra)

This doctor reflected his own knowledge of folk medicine and was incorporating it into his medical practice. Helman argues that a similar phenomenon exists in relation to advice given for colds and flu, and doctors 'give diagnoses and treatment which clearly "make sense" in the terms of reference of the folk model' (1978, p. 132). In relation to discomforts of pregnancy this knowledge appears to be the exception rather than the norm.

Women who did not have access to knowledge of traditional remedies (either because their mother or mother-in-law was dead, or living a long distance away) and those women who were sceptical of folk knowledge, were likely to be more dependent on their GP or other medical personnel. If their GP was not forthcoming with information about how to relieve the discomfort, some women would persist in asking different health workers until they received advice which was acceptable to them and alleviated the condition.

> I've had constipation . . . I did mention it at the *doctor's* once, you know. They asked if my bowels were alright and I did mention that. And I did mention it at the *hospital*. And he did say there that I could take a mild laxative if I wanted to. This was when perhaps I was about five months, but I did mention it to the *midwife* up at my doctor's and I asked her if I could take things like Andrews Liver Salts or Enos. And she said 'No don't take anything like that. Just eat more fruit and prunes – eat foods. That'll get you better – foods that'll work it out'. (Emphasis added) (Deborah)

It is interesting to note that the advice this woman eventually received was based on folk knowledge about the importance of diet for relieving discomforts. Unlike the women who tried home cures first and then sought out medical advice, she approached her doctor first and ended up using traditional recipes to alleviate the condition.

Other women often did not consult their doctor about discomforts as they felt they might be prescribed some form of medication. These women stoically suffered the discomfort because they did not believe in taking drugs whilst pregnant:

> I wouldn't take anything anyway, even if prescribed by the doctor. I'm funny like that . . . Even for sickness, if I had it, I wouldn't take anything. My sister had a lot of trouble with sickness and she was on tablets galore. She was due as now is, more or less, and she lost hers at six months. It was born normally. I don't know what the trouble is with her I'm sure, she's taken so much. She's pregnant again now, once again she's sick a lot. I said to her 'Are you taking tablets?' and she said 'No. I'm not going to bother this time'. I think it's best let alone if you can cope with it. (Mary)

> I was frightened about drugs and things. I won't even take an Aspirin or Paracetomol or anything. Sometimes I wish, if I have a bad headache or something, I wish I could take one. But I couldn't, I'm quite firm about that. (Barbara)

It was the white women who were more aware of the dangers of taking drugs in pregnancy and 38 per cent of them said that they would not take *any* drugs and would often suffer pain that they would have taken pain killers for if they had not been pregnant. Other women said they would only take medical prescriptions as a 'last resort':

> I'm not the one who likes to take pills – only as a *last resort*. I didn't take any during my first or second pregnancy. (Sabina)

Prescribers There is evidence to suggest that for many illnesses most patients consult their doctor expecting a prescription (Stimson, 1976, p. 91). As we have seen in relation to pregnancy, some doctors and women do not think that it is advisable for drugs to be taken during pregnancy. Whilst recent ideology propounds that there is a pill for every occasion (cf. Klass, 1975, p. 45), it might also be stated 'every occasion *but* pregnancy'. Women who receive medication in pregnancy therefore find themselves in the centre of a medical debate about prescribing practice in pregnancy. In the sample studied it became apparent that most of the GPs were reluctant to prescribe drugs for pregnant women; as stated before, the discomforts of pregnancy were seen to be 'normal' and 'nothing to worry about'.

The GPs who did prescribe drugs were most likely to prescribe anti-emetics to stop sickness and vomiting. Twenty-seven per cent of the women who reported suffering from sickness and vomiting to their GP were prescribed some form of medication. Only one woman however found that the tablets provided complete relief from the sickness.

> I took them and it was just – I couldn't believe the difference really . . . But it was great not being sick, I must say it was great. (Ann)

Most women only went to the GP asking for a prescription as a *last resort*, when they could no longer tolerate the sickness/vomiting. However the medical prescription did not always provide complete relief and often the women did not finish the full course of treatment.

> I used to vomit a yellowish, greenish liquid . . . I couldn't even speak for three months, then I went to the doctor. He gave me medicine, but there wasn't much difference with the medicine. But it automatically got okay after three months. (Gurmej)

> When it was Easter time as I started being sick, I realised I was pregnant and I went up to the doctor's, you know, *after so long as I could stand it.* 'Cos some nights it used to be unbearable 'cos the pains and that I got in my stomach. And um . . . he gave me some tablets, but I didn't take many, about half a dozen, because they say you don't want to have too many. You don't know what it does to the baby – there's got to be something in it. So I thought I'm not taking any more, and I just put up with it after that. (Emphasis added) (Frances)

There are two main concerns expressed in the statements given by women who did not complete the full course of prescribed treatment. These concerns were, first, a feeling that the medical treatment was not alleviating the ailment, and sometimes that it was aggravating the condition; and, second, a concern that the medical prescription might in some way harm the baby. (None of the women who used traditional recipes for these same discomforts expressed any such concern.) The anxiety about the side effects of drugs on the developing foetus, and the perceived ineffectiveness of some treatments, meant that many women stopped taking the medication.

The women often found that the treatment for sickness or vomiting and for constipation tended to aggravate the initial condition. One woman who was prescribed tablets for constipation (rather than a change in diet) said:

> I couldn't go to the toilet [embarrassed]. I did ask the doctor and he gave me something which took a long time to work, so I stopped taking it and haven't asked since. (Noleen)

Additionally, the women spoke about the adverse effects iron tablets had:

> I could never take them. If I took an iron tablet . . . it sticks, the tablet always sticks in my throat . . . So I don't take them. (Margaret)

> They [iron tablets] weren't any good, they used to make me feel sick afterwards. So I used to miss them sometimes you know. (Jaswinder)

These women mentioned to their GP that the iron tablets did not agree with them. The first woman had received iron injections in her first pregnancy and hoped to have the same in this pregnancy, but her GP did not comply with her request. The second woman told the doctor that the iron tablets made her feel sick and he changed them to some which did not have the same effect.

Neither medicines prescribed for discomforts nor those taken prophylactically (such as iron tablets) were continued by the women if they had any adverse effect. Treatment was also discontinued if the woman felt anxious about the potential effects of the drug on the foetus. The thalidomide scandal and the more recent concern expressed over Debendox (*Guardian*, 1984) made women aware of the possible harmful consequences of anti-emetic drugs.

> I don't know what they'll do, so I won't take them [pills] . . . I think it's just things published like the thalidomide, and that makes you worry. (Barbara)

The women who were least likely to take these drugs were the white middle class women who were most familiar with the publicity surrounding harmful effects of drugs in pregnancy. Certainly in the case of thalidomide, doctors had been assured of the safety of the drug Distaval which caused malformations in foetuses (Sjoström and Nilsson, 1972, p. 195). Some of the white women therefore doubted the doctor's knowledge about the safety of certain prescribed drugs.

> At the beginning of pregnancy I had a lot of migraine and he [GP] says 'These tablets are safe'. But when I got home I thought about it and I thought 'No. I'd rather not take anything because of the possible dangers, especially in the early months'. (Janice)

The women who said they would not take any drugs at all in pregnancy faced a dilemma when they suffered a painful illness. When this happened to one of the women, she consulted her doctor and was prepared to take the doctor's word that the drugs prescribed were safe.

> I had an ear infection a few weeks ago and they gave me a course of antibiotics, some ear drops and some painkillers. That set up a

> vaginal infection, with the antibiotic, so they gave me some more tablets to combat the antibiotics which were causing that. So now I'm taking about seven lots of tablets at the moment . . . He [GP] in fact got out his medical book and said 'I'm going to prescribe a new course of antibiotics, let me just check that everything's alright' . . . I'd literally taken nothing not even an Aspirin . . . I know well enough that I shouldn't so I've avoided taking anything really. (Rachel)

This dilemma was further accentuated when women suffered from an acute illness episode and were hospitalised. In these instances, women were either given drugs they would not normally have taken in pregnancy, or they found that they received medication in hospital which was subsequently denied to them on discharge.

> [When in hospital] All they did was fill me full of drugs as I said, which is something you always avoid. You don't take drugs when you're pregnant like. Everybody knows that. From the moment I was in there, I was on those tranquillisers – they've got some real good ones like, they make you sort of dizzy! (Mary, hospitalised for high blood pressure)

> They give you tablets in the hospital and when you go to your doctor, he doesn't give you none. It's funny isn't it? I suppose they don't want to take on any responsibility in case anything happens or something, perhaps that's why . . . (Wendy)

It seems as if the distinction is between being pregnant and at home under GP care, which is 'normal' and being hospitalised which is 'not normal'. One woman who suffered from sleeplessness in pregnancy worked out her own means of bridging this contradiction when she was hospitalised.

> In hospital . . . they come round and say 'Do you want any sleeping tablets?' And they give you two, and two painkillers as well, and two iron tablets – so that was six tablets I had. But I didn't take them all, I kept some for the next day, then if I had any left over I brought them home. I knew he [GP] wouldn't give me none over the road, so I kept 'em. (Sheilagh)

Managing to obtain symptomatic relief for some women was a matter of constant negotiation with their doctor and the white women tended to be more skilful in this because they have greater experience of the health service in Britain. White women, as mentioned above, also tended to be more sceptical of the 'safety' of drugs and to have more knowledge of their potentially harmful consequences.

Conclusion

Pregnancy is neither a pathological state as depicted by some members of the medical profession, nor an idealised state of harmony with nature. The reality of pregnancy for most women is that they feel positively about their health, while at the same time suffering from discomforts which they seek to alleviate.

The medical profession appears inadequate in dealing with the discomforts of pregnancy. This may be related to two factors. First, the complaints of pregnant women are not taken seriously, in the same way that other 'feminine' complaints to do with reproduction are often regarded as trivial (Elston, 1981). They are either seen to be psychogenic in origin and therefore not warranting symptomatic relief, or they are viewed as a 'normal' part of pregnancy and something that pregnant women must endure. Second, the medical profession is caught in a considerable dilemma about the prescription of drugs in pregnancy, particularly for discomforts and, as we have seen in this study, GPs do tend to fall into the two distinct camps of 'prescribers' and 'non-prescribers'.

If doctors are going to be active in alleviating suffering caused by minor illnesses such as the discomforts of pregnancy, then they need to take these conditions more seriously and perhaps consider non-pharmaceutical ways of easing suffering, while at the same time recognising that home remedies may provide effective symptomatic relief in some cases. They could thus learn from women's traditional knowledge of healing and reinforce this knowledge rather than undermining it as 'old wives' tales'. Moreover they need to listen to what women say about their social circumstances and how these are affecting their experience of pregnancy.

Women themselves have different ways of dealing with discomforts and this relates to their class and cultural background together with the strength of their lay support system (particularly the support of older knowledgeable women). For white women the differences in dealing with discomforts of pregnancy are closely related to social class; working class women in the first instance will try traditional recipes and home cures, while the middle class women are most likely to consult their GP as a first resort.

Elsewhere I have shown that Punjabi women draw on a wealth of knowledge about health maintenance during pregnancy (Homans, 1983) and this chapter refers to their knowledge of home remedies for alleviating discomforts. This knowledge forms part of a coherent philosophy which stresses the importance of diet in maintaining and restoring health. In the absence of an older female relative to impart this knowledge, and in cases where symptoms persist, western medical treatment is sought. However, Punjabi women in this situation may not have knowledge about possible siue effects of medication during pregnancy and be more dependent on the doctor and on what is prescribed. This has to be seen in the context of what happens to populations on migration and how traditional knowledge and social support networks are broken down. Additionally, there is always pressure on immigrant groups to adapt to the ways of the 'host' population and in the context of health care there are educational programmes to encourage black and ethnic minority populations to consult doctors in the first instance and not to use their home remedies. This is part of a process in which western medicine undermines folk knowledge and home cures and denies the validity of women's healing qualities.

The undermining of Punjabi women's healing qualities tends to make the women more dependent on the medical profession who, as we have seen, offer little constructive help with the discomforts of pregnancy. This is certainly happening to women who do not have older female relatives at hand; such women consult their GP as a first resort and tend to accept the medication prescribed. It is therefore foreseeable that Punjabi women will use western medicine more, at a time when some white women are becoming more questioning about antenatal care in general and about drugs and technological interventions in particular. There is a move by some white women to recover traditional healing skills and the curative properties of home remedies.

Finally, this discussion of discomforts in pregnancy should be seen in the context of individualised antenatal care in Britain which, together with the racism present in British society, ensures that there is no forum for women to meet together and discuss the sorts of issues that have been raised in this chapter. White women could certainly learn much from Punjabi women about home remedies while in turn, Punjabi women may want more information about the potentially harmful effects of certain drugs in pregnancy. The challenge for us is therefore to break down these barriers and share our knowledge with all women, irrespective of their race and social class. Through this process we will learn more about our bodies and how to maintain and restore health, at the same time as creating a support network for us all.

Notes

1. Seventy-seven per cent of the Asian women in the final sample were born in the Punjab. Of the Gujerati women in the sample, one was born in Britain, one came to Britain straight from Gujerat, one via Tanzania and one via Kenya. Two women had migrated from Pakistan. Sixty-five per cent of these women had lived in the city for less than six years; by comparison, eighty-five per cent of the white women had lived in the city all their lives.

   The difficulties of ascribing social class to women are numerous and for the purposes of this chapter social class is used to reflect the women's social status and access to material resources (Homans, 1980, pp. 211–7). Using this classification forty-two per cent of the white women were middle class, while the Asian women were, with one exception, working class.

2. None of the publications given out at the antenatal clinic or the parentcraft classes were in any of the Asian languages, yet eleven per cent of births in the city were to Asian women who did not have English as their first language. The first languages of the women in the sample were Punjabi (69 per cent), Gujerati (23 per cent) and Urdu (8 per cent).

Acknowledgements

My thanks are due to Bhupinder Dhesi who proved an invaluable interpreter and also gave an insight into Punjabi culture; and to the Birmingham Interpreting and Translating Service for translation and transcription of tapes. Finally, I would particularly like to thank all the women who participated in the study and gave their time and shared their knowledge so generously.

Bibliography

Aitken-Swan, J. (1977) *Fertility Control and the Medical Profession*, London, Croom Helm.

Alberman, E. and Berry, A.C. (1979) 'Prenatal diagnosis and the specialist in community medicine', *Community Medicine*, vol. 1, 89–96.

Alberman, E., Berry, A.C. and Polani, P.E. (1979) 'Planning an amniocentesis service for Down's syndrome', *Lancet*, vol. 1, 50.

Alberman, E. and Dennis, K.J. (ed.) (1984) *Late Abortions in England and Wales*, London, Royal College of Obstetrics and Gynaecology.

Allen, I. (1981) *Family Planning, Sterilization and Abortion Services*, London, Policy Studies Institute.

Ardener, S. (ed.) (1981) *Women and Space: Ground Rules and Social Maps*, London, Croom Helm.

Arditti, R., Duelli Klein, R. and Minden, S. (1984) *Test-tube Women: What Future for Motherhood?*, London, Pandora Press.

Armstrong, D. (n.d.) *Pathological Life and Death: Medical Spatialisation and Geriatrics*. Mimeo from Department of Community Medicine, Guy's Hospital, London.

Ashton, J.R. (1980) 'Components of delay amongst women obtaining a termination of pregnancy', *Journal of Biosocial Science*, vol. 12, part 3, 261–273.

Association for Improvements in the Maternity Services (1983) 'The unknowns of ultrasound', *Aims Quarterly Journal*, Summer issue, 15.

Austin, C. (1974) 'Recent progress in the study of eggs and spermatozoa: Insemination and ovulation to implantation', in A. Guyton and G. Horobin (eds), *Reproductive Physiology*, Series 1, vol. 8, MIT International Review of Science, 95–131.

Baldwin, S. and Glendinning, C. (1983) 'Employment, women and their disabled children', in J. Finch and G. Groves (eds), *A Labour of Love: Women, Work and Caring*, London, Routledge and Kegan Paul, 53–71.

Barker-Benfield, B. (1976) *The Horrors of the Half-known Life, Male Attitudes towards Woman and Sexuality in Nineteenth Century America*, New York, Harper and Row, 80–132.

Barnes, J. (1976) *Essentials of Family Planning*, Oxford, Blackwell Scientific Publications.

Barrett, M. and Roberts, H. (1978) 'Doctors and their patients: the social control of women in general practice', in C. Smart and B. Smart (eds), *Women, Sexuality and Social Control*, London, Routledge and Kegan Paul, 41–52.

Barth, F. (1969) *Ethnic Groups and Boundaries*, Boston, Little Brown.

de Beauvoir, S. (1972) *The Second Sex*, Harmondsworth, Penguin Books.

Beckett, S. (1973) *Herbs for Feminine Ailments*, Thornson.

Begley, D.J., Firth, J.A. and Hoult, J.R.S. (1980) *Human Reproduction and Developmental Biology*, London, Macmillan.

Benson, R.C. (1972) 'Gynaecology and obstetrics', in M.J. Krupp and M.J. Chatton (eds), *Current Medical Diagnosis and Treatment*, Los Altos, California, Lange Medical Publications, 377–434.

Birke, L. and Best, S. (1980) 'The tyrannical womb: menstruation and menopause', in Brighton Women and Science Group (ed.), *Alice through the Microscope. The Power of Science over Women's Lives*, London, Virago, 89–107.

Birkett Committee (1939) *Report of the Inter-departmental Committee on Abortion*, Ministry of Health, Home Office, London, HMSO.

Birth Control Trust (1984) *Men, Sex and Contraception*, London, Family Planning Association.

Bishop, W.H. and Walton, A. (1956) 'Spermatogenesis and the structure of mammalian spermatozoon', in A.S. Parkes (ed.), *Marshall's Physiology of Reproduction*, London, Longmans, vol. 1, part 2, 1–101.

Bland, L. *et al.* (1978) 'Women "inside and outside" the relations of production', in Women's Studies Group, Centre for Contemporary Cultural Studies, University of Birmingham (ed.), *Women Take Issue. Aspects of Women's Subordination*, London, Hutchinson.

Blum, R. and Kreitman, K. (1981) 'Factors affecting individual use of medicines', in R. Blum *et al.* (eds), *Pharmaceuticals and Health Policy*, London, Croom Helm, 122–185.

Blum, R., Herxheimer, A., Stenzl, C. and Woodcock, J. (eds) (1981) *Pharmaceuticals and Health Policy*, London, Croom Helm.

Bone, M. (1973) *The Family Planning Services in England and Wales*, London, DHSS, HMSO.

Bone, M. (1978) *The Family Planning Services: Changes and Effects*, London, DHSS, HMSO.

Bowlby, J. (1952) *Maternal Care and Maternal Health*, Geneva, World Health Organisation, Monograph Series No. 2.

Bradbury, M. (1977) *The History Man*, London, Arrow Books.

Bradshaw, J. (1982) 'Now what are they up to? Men in the "Men's Movement"', in S. Friedman and E. Sarah (eds), *On the Problem of Men*, London, The Women's Press, 174–189.

British Medical Association (1936) *Report of Committee on Medical Aspects of Abortion*.

British Medical Association (1975) *You and Your Baby, Part 1, From Pregnancy to Birth*, London, A Family Doctor Publication.

British Medical Journal (1958) answer to a question about oral contraception, vol. 2, 1116.

British Medical Journal (1971) 'Abortion or contraception?', vol. 3, 261–262.

British Medical Journal (1972) Leading Article, 'Doctors and population', vol. 1, 391.

British Medical Journal (1973) Leading Article, 'The case for free contraceptives', vol. 1, 130.

British Medical Journal (1976) Leading Article, 'Contraceptive dynamism', vol. 2, 1405–1406.

British Medical Journal (1977) 'Diagnostic amniocentesis in early pregnancy', 4 June, 1430–1431.

British Medical Journal (1978) 'Hazards of amniocentesis', vol. 2, 1661–1662.

British Medical Journal (1979) Leading Article, 'Tomorrow's contraceptive: yesterday's problem?', vol. 2, 951.

British Pregnancy Advisory Service (1978) *Abortion Today*, London, BPAS.

Brown, J. (1970) 'A note on the division of labor by sex', *American Anthropologist*, vol. 72, 1073–1078.

Browner, C. and Lewin, E. (1982) 'Female altruism reconsidered: the Virgin Mary as economic woman', *American Ethnologist*, vol. 9, no. 1, 61–75.

Bruhn, J.A. and Parsons, O.A. (1964) 'Medical student attitudes toward four medical specialties', *Journal of Medical Education*, vol. 39, 40–49.

Campbell, S. (1979) 'Window in the womb', *Action Magazine*, Spring issue, 15–18.

Carby, H.V. (1982) 'White woman listen! Black feminism and the boundaries of sisterhood', in Centre for Contemporary Cultural Studies (eds), *The Empire Strikes Back: Race and Racism in 70s Britain*, London, Hutchinson, 212–235.

Cartwright, A. (1976) 'What goes on in the general practitioner's surgery?', in R.M. Acheson and L. Aird (eds), *Seminar in Community Medicine*, vol. 1 Sociology, Oxford, Oxford University Press.

Cartwright, A. (1978) *Recent Trends in Family Building and Contraception*, London, OPCS, HMSO.

Cartwright, A. (1979) *The Dignity of Labour*, London, Tavistock.

Centre for Contemporary Cultural Studies (eds) (1982) *The Empire Strikes Back: Race and Racism in 70s Britain*, London, Hutchinson.

Chacko, A. (1982) 'Too many daughters? India's drastic cure', *World Paper*, November, 8–9.

Chamberlain, M. (1981) *Old Wives' Tales: Their History, Remedies and Spells*, London, Virago.

Chard, T. and Richards, M.P.M. (eds) (1977) *Benefits and Hazards of the New Obstetrics*, London, Heinemann Medical Books.

CHC News (1978) 'Spina bifida screening', May, 6, 7, 11.

Chesser, E. (1949) *Society and Abortion*, London, Abortion Law Reform Association.

Chester, R. and Peel, J. (eds) (1977) *Equalities and Inequalities in Family Life*, London, Academic Press.

Chodorow, N. (1974) 'Family structure and feminine personality', in M.Z. Rosaldo and L. Lamphere (eds), *Woman, Culture and Society*, Stanford, CA, Stanford University Press, 43–66.

Christopher, E. (1980) *Sexuality and Birth Control in Social and Community Work*, London, Temple Smith.

Clinical Genetics Society (1978) *The Provision of Services for the Prenatal Diagnosis of Foetal Abnormality in the United Kingdom*, London, The Eugenics Society.

Conrad, P. (1984) book review, *Observer*, 8 April.

Co-ord, (1981) 'What is Co-ord?' Co-ord: 27–35 Mortimer Street, London, W.1.

Cossey, D. (1979) *The Case for the Condom*, London, Brook Advisory Centres.

Curie-Cohen, M., Luttrell, L. and Shapiro, S. (1979) 'Current practices of artificial insemination by donor in the United States', *New England Journal of Medicine*, vol. 300, no. 11, 585–590.

Daily Express (1977) 'A step nearer the day when every baby is born healthy', 8 December.

Daly, M. (1978) *Gyn/ecology: The Metaethics of Radical Feminism*, London, Women's Press.

Davies, T.B. *et al.* (1939) *The Queen Charlotte's Text Book of Obstetrics*, London, J. & A. Churchill Ltd.

Davin, A. (1978) 'Imperialism and motherhood', *History Workshop Journal*, vol. 5, Spring, 9–65.

Davis, A. (1950) *British Medical Journal*, vol. 2, 123–130.

Davis, A. (1982) *Women, Race and Class*, London, The Women's Press. (First published in the United States by Random House, 1981.)

Day, P. (1982) *Women Doctors. Choices and Constraints in Policies for Medical Manpower*, a study commissioned by King Edward's Hospital Fund for London, London, Kings Fund Centre.

Day, S. (1982) 'Is obstetric technology depressing?', *Radical Science Journal*, no. 12, 17–45.

Deutsch, H. (1944) *The Psychology of Women. A Psychoanalytic Interpretation*, London, Heinemann.

Dewhurst, J. and Scott, J.S. (1978) 'Spina bifida children', *Times*, 14 February.

DHSS (1976a) *Prevention and Health: Everybody's Business*, London, HMSO.

DHSS (1976b) *Priorities for Health and Personal Services in England*, London, HMSO.

DHSS (1977a) *Reducing the Risk: Safer Pregnancy and Childbirth*, London, HMSO.

DHSS (1979a) *Report by the Working Group on Screening for Neural Tube Defects*, London, DHSS.

DHSS (1979b) *Report on Confidential Enquiries into Maternal Deaths in England and Wales 1973–75*, Table 5.7, London, HMSO.

Donald, I. (1980) 'Hereditary disease: the real need to know more', *Action Magazine*, Spring issue, 23–27.

Donovan, J. (1983), 'Black people's health: a different way forward?', *Radical Community Medicine*, Winter, 20–29.

Doyal, L. with Pennell, I. (1979) *The Political Economy of Health*, London, Pluto Press.

Dubin, L. and Amelar, R.D. (1980) 'A plea for a more scientific approach in the treatment of male fertility', *Fertility and Sterility*, vol. 34, no. 1, 74–75.

Duelli Klein, R. (1984) 'Doing it ourselves: self-insemination', in R. Arditti *et al.* (eds), *Test-tube Women: What Future for Motherhood?*, London, Pandora Press, 382–390.

Dumont, L. (1970) *Homo Hierarchicus: The Caste System and its Implications*, Chicago, University of Chicago Press.

Dunnell, K. (1979) *Family Formation 1976*, Office of Population Censuses and Surveys, London, HMSO.

Dunnell, K. and Cartwright, A. (1972) *Medicine Takers, Hoarders and Prescribers*, London, Routledge and Kegan Paul.

Eaton, G. and Parish, P. (1976) 'Medical training and prescribing activity', in P.A. Parish *et al.*, Prescribing in general practice, *Journal of the Royal College of General Practitioners*, vol. 26, no. 1, 31–34.

Edholm, F., Harris, O. and Young, K. (1977) 'Conceptualising women', *Critique of Anthropology*, vol. 3, 101–130.

Edinburgh Sunday Standard (1981), 24th May.

Ehrenreich, B. (1974) 'Gender and objectivity in medicine', *International Journal of Health Services*, vol. 4, part 4, 617–623.

Ehrenreich, B. and English, D. (1973) *Complaints and Disorders: The Sexual Politics of Sickness*, London, Compendium.

Ehrenreich, B. and English, D. (1978) *For Her Own Good: 150 Years of the Experts' Advice to Women*, New York, Anchor Press.

Elston, M.A. (1977) 'Women in the medical profession: whose problem?', in M. Stacey *et al.* (eds), *Health and the Division of Labour*, London, Croom Helm, 115–140.

Elston, M.A. (1981) 'Medicine as "old husbands' tales": the impact of feminism', in D. Spender (ed.), *Men's Studies Modified*, Oxford, Pergamon, 189–211.

Elston, M.A. and Doyal, L. (1983) 'Health and medicine', Unit 14, Course no. U221, *The Changing Experience of Women*, Milton Keynes, Open University Press.

Enkin, M. and Chalmers, I. (1982) *Effectiveness and Satisfaction in Ante-natal Care*, London, Heinemann Medical Books.

Entwistle, D.R. and Doering, S.G. (1981) *The First Birth: A Family Turning Point*, Baltimore, Johns Hopkins University Press.

Evening News (1978) January.

Fabe, M. and Wikler, N. (1979) *Up Against the Clock*, New York, Random House.

Faithorn, E. (1975) 'The concept of pollution among the kafe of the Papua New Guinea Highlands', in R. Reiter (ed.), *Toward an Anthropology of Women*, New York, Monthly Review Press, 127–140.

Farrant, W. (1980a) 'Stress after amniocentesis for high serum alpha-fetoprotein concentration', *British Medical Journal*, vol. 281, 452.

Farrant, W. (1980b) 'Importance of counselling in ante-natal screening', *MIMS Magazine*, 15 June, 55–63.

Farrant, W. (1983) 'Prenatal screening (Part 1) – overlooking women's needs', *Maternity Action*, 9, 4–5.

Farrant, W. (1983) 'Prenatal screening (Part 2) – an agenda for better practice', *Maternity Action*, 10, 5 and 11.

Farrell, C. in collaboration with Kellaher, L. (1978) *My Mother Said . . . The Way Young People Learned about Sex and Birth Control*, London, Routledge and Kegan Paul.

Fawcett, D. (1977) 'The structure of the spermatozoon' in Greep *et al.* (eds), *Frontiers in Reproduction and Fertility Control*, London, MIT Press, 353–378.

Fawcett, D. (1979) 'The cell biology of gametogenesis in the male', *Perspectives in Biology and Medicine*, Winter 1979, Part 2, S56–S73.

Finch, J. and Groves, D. (eds) (1983) *A Labour of Love: Women, Work and Caring*, London, Routledge and Kegan Paul.

Finegold, W. (1964) *Artificial Insemination*, Springfield, IL, Charles C. Thomas.

Finger, A. (1984) 'Claiming all of our bodies: reproductive rights and disabilities', in R. Arditti *et al.* (eds), *Test-tube Women: What Future for Motherhood?*, London, Pandora Press, 281–297.

Fisher, S. (1984) 'Doctor–patient communication: a social and micro-political performance', *Sociology of Health and Illness*, vol. 6, no. 1, 1–29.

Foster, G. (1961) 'The dyadic contract: a model for the social structure of a Mexican peasant village', *American Anthropologist*, vol. 65, 1173–1192.

Foster, G. (1963) 'The dyadic contract in Tzintzuntzan, II: patron–client relationships', *American Anthropologist*, vol. 65, 1280–1294.

Frankl, G. (1975) *The Failure of the Sexual Revolution*, London, New English Library.

Freidson, E. (1960) 'Client control and medical practice', *American Journal of Sociology*, vol. 65, January, 374–382.

Freund, M. (1966) 'Standards for the rating of human sperm morphology', *International Journal of Fertility*, vol. 11, no. 1, part 2, January–March, 97–119.

Friberg, J. and Gemzell, C. (1977) 'Sperm-freezing and donor insemination', *International Journal of Fertility*, vol. 22, no. 3, 148–154.

Galtung, J. (1967) *Theory and Methods of Social Research*, London, Allen and Unwin.

Garcia, J. (1982) 'Women's views of ante-natal care', in M. Elkin and I. Chalmers (eds), *Effectiveness and Satisfaction in Ante-natal Care*, London, Heinemann Medical Books, 81–91.

Garland, G.W., Quixley, J.M.E. and Cameron, M.D. (1976) *Obstetrics and Gynaecology for Nurses*, London, Hodder and Stoughton Educational (3rd edition).

Gifford, P.W. (1971) Letter to *British Medical Journal*, vol. 3, 534.

Gifford, P.W., Guillebaud, J., Collcutt, E. and Francis, G.M. (1971) Letter to *British Medical Journal*, vol. 3, 584.

Glass, N. (1976) *Economic Consequences for the Public Sector of a Spina Bifida Screening Programme*, DHSS Economic Adviser's Office.

Gordon, L. (1977) *Woman's Body, Woman's Right*, Harmondsworth, Penguin Books.

Goshen-Gottstein, E. (1966) *Marriage and First Pregnancy*, London, Tavistock Publications.

Graham, H. (1977a) 'Images of pregnancy in ante-natal literature', in R. Dingwall *et al.* (eds), *Health Care and Health Knowledge*, London, Croom Helm, 15–37.

Graham, H. (1977b) 'Women's attitudes to conception and pregnancy', in R. Chester and J. Peel (eds), *Equalities and Inequalities in Family Life*, London, Academic Press, 81–97.

Graham, H. (1980) 'Prevention and health: every mother's business: a comment on child health policy in the 1970s', in C.C. Harris (ed.), *The Sociology of the Family: New Directions for Britain*, Keele, Sociological Review Monograph, 160–185.

Graham, H. (1984a) 'Providers, negotiators and mediators: women as the hidden carers', in E. Lewin and V. Olesen (eds), *Women, Health and Healing: Toward a New Perspective*, London/New York, Tavistock/Methuen (forthcoming).

Graham, H. (1984b) *Women, Health and the Family*, Brighton, Wheatsheaf Books.

Graham, H. and Oakley, A. (1981) 'Competing ideologies of reproduction – medical and maternal perspectives on pregnancy', in H. Roberts (ed.), *Women, Health and Reproduction*, London, Routledge and Kegan Paul, 50–74.

Grant, J.M. and Hussein, I.Y. (1984) 'An audit of abdominal hysterectomy over a decade in a district hospital', *British Journal of Obstetrics and Gynaecology*, vol. 91, January, 73–77.

Greenwood, V. and Young, J. (1976) *Abortion on Demand*, London, Pluto Press.

Guardian (1978) 'Specialists disagree over spina bifida screening', 9 January.

Guardian (1984) 'Firm in birth defects dispute to pay $120m', 16 July.

Guillebaud, J. (1975) Letter to *British Medical Journal*, vol. 1, 457.

Hagard, S. and Carter, F.A. (1976) 'Preventing the birth of infants with Down's syndrome', *British Medical Journal*, vol. 1, 753–756.

Hagard, S., Carter, F.A. and Milne, R.G. (1976) 'Screening for spina bifida cystica: A cost benefit analysis', *British Journal of Preventive and Social Medicine*, vol. 30, no. 1, 40–53.

Haire, D. (1972) *The Cultural Warping of Childbirth*, International Childbirth Education Association News.

Hampson, K. (1978) 'Putting the rights of every expectant mother to the test', *Guardian*, 22 March.

Hanmer, J. (1981) 'Sex predetermination and male dominance', in H. Roberts (ed.), *Women, Health and Reproduction*, London, Routledge and Kegan Paul, 163–190.

Harris, C.M. (1981) 'Medical stereotypes', *British Medical Journal*, vol. 283, 19–26 December, 1676–1677.

Harrison, N. (1979) *Infertility*, Boston, Houghton Mifflin.

Hearn, K. (1983) 'The right to life', *In from the Cold*, no. 7, Summer, 14–15.

Helman, C.G. (1978) 'Feed a cold, starve a fever: folk models of infection in an English suburban community and their relation to medical treatment',

Culture, Medicine and Psychiatry, vol. 2, 107–137.

Hern, W. (1971) 'Is pregnancy really normal?', *Family Planning Perspectives*, vol. 3, January, 5–10.

Hern, W. (1975) 'The illness parameters of pregnancy', *Social Science and Medicine*, vol. 9, 365.

Herschberger, R. (1970) *Adam's Rib*, New York, Harper and Row.

Herxheimer, A. and Stimson, G. (1981) 'The use of medicines for illness', in R. Blum *et al.* (eds), *Pharmaceuticals and Health Policy*, London, Croom Helm, 36–60.

Hindell, K. and Simms, M. (1971) *Abortion Law Reformed*, London, Peter Owen.

Hite, S. (1981) *The Hite Report on Male Sexuality*, London, MacDonald.

HMSO (1934) 'On the state of the public health: Annual report to the Chief Medical Officer of the Ministry of Health', 1933.

HMSO (1967) Abortion Act.

Hoffman, L.W. (1978) 'Effects of the first child on the woman's role', in W.B. Miller and L.F. Newman (eds), *The First Child and Family Formation*, Chapel Hill, Carolina Population Center, 340–367.

Holterman, S. (1977) *Costs of Screening Programme for Neural Tube Defects*, DHSS Economic Adviser's Office.

Homans, H. (1980) 'Pregnant in Britain: a sociological approach to Asian and British women's experiences', University of Warwick, unpublished PhD thesis, July.

Homans, H. (1982) 'Pregnancy and birth as "rites of passage" for two groups of women in Britain', in C.P. MacCormack (ed.), *Ethnography of Fertility and Birth*, London, Academic Press, 231–268.

Homans, H. (1983) 'A question of balance: Asian and British women's perception of food during pregnancy', in A. Murcott (ed.), *The Sociology of Food and Eating*, Aldershot, Gower, 73–83.

Homans, H. and Satow, A. (1981) 'We are strangers too. Cultural concepts of health and illness', *Journal of Community Nursing*, November, 10–13.

Homans, H. and Satow, A. (1982) 'Can you hear me? Cultural variations in communication', *Journal of Community Nursing*, January, 16–18.

Hooks, B. (1981) *Ain't I a woman: black women and feminism*, London, Pluto Press.

Hornstein, F. (1984) 'Children by donor insemination: a new choice for lesbians', in R. Arditti *et al.* (eds), *Test-tube women: what future motherhood?*, London, Pandora, 373–390.

Hoskins, B.B. and Holmes, H.B. (1984) 'Technology and prenatal femicide', in R. Arditti *et al.* (eds), *Test-tube women: what future motherhood?*, London, Pandora, 237–255.

House of Commons (1980) *Perinatal and Neonatal Mortality*, Second report for the Social Services Committee, House of Commons paper 663–1 (session 1979–80), London, HMSO.

House of Commons Debates (1980) vol. 992, no. 244, part 1, columns 258–260.

House of Commons Debates (1981) *National Health Service Act 1977* (Amendment), vol. 7, no. 132, columns 877–882.

House of Commons Debates (1982a) vol. 21, no. 88, column 90.

House of Commons Debates (1982b) vol. 22, no. 100, column 101.

House of Lords Debates (1967) vol. 285, no. 188, columns 1426–35.

Hubbard, R. (1981) 'The Emperor doesn't wear any clothes: the impact of feminism in biology', in D. Spender (ed.), *Men's Studies Modified*, Oxford, Pergamon, 213–235.

Hudson, B., Baker, H.W.G. and de Kretser, D.M. (1980) 'The abnormal semen sample', in R.J. Pepperell, B. Hudson and C. Wood (eds), *The Infertile Couple*, New York, Churchill Livingstone, 70–111.

Hudson, B. and Burger, H. (1979) 'Physiology and function of the testes', in P. Shearman (ed.), *Human Reproductive Physiology*, Oxford, Blackwell, 73–96.

Humphreys, C. (1979) 'Disability in Britain today', *Medicine in Society*, vol. 5, no. 1, 8–13.

Hunter, N.D. and Polikoff, N.D. (1976) 'Custody rights of lesbian mothers: legal theory and litigation strategy', *Buffalo Law Review*, vol. 25, 691–733.

International Planned Parenthood Federation (1980) *Family Planning Handbook for Doctors* (5th edn), R.L. Kleinman (ed.), London, International Planned Parenthood Federation Publications.

Jackson, S. (1980) 'Girls and sexual knowledge', in D. Spender and E. Sarah (eds), *Learning to Lose: Sexism and Education*, London, The Women's Press, 131–145.

Jackson, S. (1982) 'Femininity, masculinity and sexuality', in S. Friedman and E. Sarah (eds), *On the Problem of Men*, London, The Women's Press, 21–28.

Jeffery, R. and Jeffery, P. (1983) 'Female infanticide and amniocentesis', *Economic and Political Weekly*, vol. 18, nos. 16–17, 16–23 April, 655–657.

Jones, B.F.S. (1952) Letter to *British Medical Journal*, vol. 1, 1027.

Kaplan, A. (1964) *The Conduct of Inquiry*, San Francisco, Chandler.

Kitzinger, S. (1978) *Women as Mothers*, Glasgow, Fontana.

Klass, A. (1975) *There's Gold in Them Thar Pills*, Harmondsworth, Penguin Books.

Lane Committee (1974) *Report of the Committee on the Working of the Abortion Act*, London, HMSO (Cmnd. 5579).

Langford, C.M. (1976) *Birth Control Practice and Marital Fertility in Great Britain*, London, Population Investigation Committee.

Larned, D. (1974) 'The greening of the womb', *New Times*, 27 December, 36.

Law, B. (1971) 'Gynaecology in general practice: methods of contraception', *British Medical Journal*, vol. 1, 444.

Laws, S. (1983a) 'Ban VAT on sanitary wear campaign', unpublished paper, Warwick University.

Laws, S. (1983b) 'The sexual politics of PMT', *Women's Studies International Quarterly*, vol. 6, no. 1, 19–31.

Laws, S. with Hey, V. (1985) *Seeing Red: the politics of premenstrual tension*, Explorations in Feminism Series, London, Hutchinson.

Leathard, A. (1980) *The Fight for Family Planning*, London, Macmillan.

Ledward, R.S., Crawford, L. and Symonds, E.M. (1979) 'Social factors in patients for artificial insemination by donor (AID)', *Journal of Biosocial Science*, vol. 11, 473–479.

Leeson, J. and Gray, J. (1978) *Women and Medicine*, London, Tavistock.

Lennane, K. and R.J. (1973) 'Alleged psychogenic disorders in women: a possible manifestation of sexual prejudice', *New England Journal of Medicine*, vol. 288, 6 February, 288–292.

Lever, J. (1979) *Premenstrual Tension: the Unrecognised Illness*, London, New English Library.

Lewin, E. (1974) *Mothers and Children: Latin American Immigrants in San Francisco*, doctoral dissertation, Stanford University.

Lewin, E. (1981) 'Lesbianism and motherhood: implications for child custody', *Human Organization*, vol. 40, no. 1, 6–14.

Lewis, J. (1980) *The Politics of Motherhood: Child and Maternal Welfare in England, 1900–1939*, London, Croom Helm.

Lewis, T.L.T. (1980) 'Legal abortion in England and Wales 1968–1978', *British Medical Journal*, vol. 1, 295–296.

Lindenbaum, S. (1972) 'Sorcerers, ghosts and polluting women: an analysis of religious belief and population control', *Ethnology*, vol. 11, no. 3, 241–253.

Lipshultz, L.T. (1982) 'Beyond the routine semen analysis', *Fertility and Sterility*, vol. 38, no. 2, 153–155.
Littlefield, J.W., Milunsky, A. and Jacoby, L.B. (1973) 'Prenatal genetic diagnosis: status and problems', in B. Hilton, D. Callahan, M. Harris, P. Condliffe and B. Berkeley (eds), *Ethical Issues in Human Genetics*, New York, Plenum Press.
MacCormack, C.P. (ed.) (1982) *Ethnography of Fertility and Birth*, London, Academic Press.
Macfarlane-Burnett, I.B. (1973) *Genes, Dreams and Realities*, Harmondsworth, Penguin Books.
Macintyre, S. (1975) *Decision-making Process following Premarital Conception*, PhD thesis, University of Aberdeen.
Macintyre, S. (1976) 'Who wants babies: the social construction of "instincts"', in D.L. Barker and S. Allen (eds), *Sexual Divisions and Society: Process and Change*, London, Tavistock, 150–179.
Macintyre, S. (1978) *Register of Research in the Sociology of Human Reproduction*, Aberdeen, Medical Research Council Unit.
Mackay, E. (1972) Letter to *British Medical Journal*, vol. 1, 244.
Mackeith, N. (ed.) (1978) *The New Women's Health Handbook*, London, Virago.
Mackintosh, M. (1977) 'Reproduction and patriarchy: A critique of Claude Meillassoux "Femmes, Greniers et Capitaux"', *Capital and Class*, Bulletin of socialist economists, Summer, 119–127.
Macnicol, J. (1980) *The Movement for Family Planning Allowances, 1918–45: A Study in Social Policy Development*, London, Heinemann.
Malleson, J. (1952) Letter to *British Medical Journal*, vol. 1, 970.
Mann, T. (1977) 'Semen: Metabolism, antigenicity, storage and artificial insemination', in Greep *et al.* (eds) *Frontiers in Reproduction and Fertility Control*, London, MIT Press, 427–433.
Marieskind, H. (1975) 'Restructuring Ob-Gyn', *Social Policy*, September/October, 48–49.
Marieskind, H. (1980) *Women in the Health System, Patients, Providers and Programs*, St Louis, C.V. Mosby Company.
Mason, M. (1981) 'Euthanasia', *In from the Cold*, no. 2, October, 11–14.
Mason, M. (1982) 'Life: whose right to choose?', *Spare Rib*, no. 115, 26.
Mason, M. (1983) 'The eugenic implications of the medical approach to disability', *Politics of Health*, no. 6, 10.
Mass, B. (1976) *Population Target: The Political Economy of Population Control in Latin America*, Toronto, The Latin American Working Group.
Maternity Alliance (1982) *It All Depends Where you Live: A Survey of Screening for Congenital Abormalities*, London, Maternity Alliance.
Medical Research Council (1978) 'An assessment of the hazards of amniocentesis', *British Journal of Obstetrics and Gynaecology*, vol. 85, supplement no. 2.
Medical Women's Federation (1952) 'Memorandum on family planning with particular reference to contraception', *British Medical Journal*, vol. 1, 595–597.
Meredith, P. (1982) *Pharmacy, Contraception and the Health Care Role*, Family Planning Association, Project Report no. 3, London.
Merrison Committee (1979) *Report of Royal Commission on the National Health Service*, London, HMSO, Cmnd 7615.
Middleton, A. (1982) 'An endangered species – feminist ethnography in a rural setting', paper presented at a meeting of the British Sociological Association's Study Group, University of Manchester, 23–24 January.
Mitchell, J. and Wilson, A. (1981) *Black People and the Health Service*, London, Brent Community Health Council.

Mozans, H.T. (1974) *Woman in Science*, London, MIT Press. (First published 1913.)

National Medical Consultative Committee (1980) *Report of the Working Party on a Maternal Serum AFP Screening Programme*, Scottish Home and Health Department.

Nelson, C.M.K. and Bunge, R.G. (1974) 'Semen analysis, evidence for changing parameters of male fertility potential', *Fertility and Sterility*, vol. 25, no. 6, 503–507.

Newton, N. (1955) *Maternal Emotions: A Study of Women's Feelings towards Menstruation, Pregnancy, Childbirth, Breast Feeding and Other Aspects of their Femininity*, New York, P.B. Hoeber.

Nichter, M. (1977) 'Health ideologies and medical cultures in the South Kanara Areca nut belt', University of Edinburgh, unpublished PhD thesis.

Nicholas, S. and Nicolas, P. (1957) Letter to *British Medical Journal*, vol. 2, 52.

Norbeck, E. (1977) 'A sanction for authority: etiquette', in R.D. Fogelson and R.N. Adams (eds) *The Anthropology of Power*, New York, Academic Press, 67–76.

North East Thames Regional Health Authority (1979) *Prenatal Screening*, April.

Notley, R. (1979) 'Transurethral resection of the prostate', *British Journal of Sexual Medicine*, July, 10–26.

Oakley, A. (1975) 'The trap of medicalised motherhood', *New Society*, 18 December, 639–641.

Oakley, A. (1976a) *Bibliography on the Sociology of Human Reproduction*, University of London, Bedford College, October.

Oakley, A. (1976b) 'Wisewoman and medicine man: changes in the management of childbirth', in J. Mitchell and A. Oakley (eds), *The Rights and Wrongs of Women*, Harmondsworth, Penguin Books, 17–58.

Oakley, A. (1982) 'The origins and development of ante-natal care', in M. Enkin and I. Chalmers (eds), *Effectiveness and Satisfaction in Ante-natal Care*, London, Heinemann Medical Books, 1–21.

O'Brien, M. (1981) *The Politics of Reproduction*, London, Routledge and Kegan Paul.

Office of Population Censuses and Surveys (1976) *Mortality Statistics 1976*, Table DH_2, London, HMSO.

Office of Population Censuses and Surveys (1974–1979) *Abortion Statistics 1974–1979*. Series AB 1, 2, 3, 4, 5, London, HMSO.

Office of Population Censuses and Surveys (1981) *Abortion Statistics*, London, HMSO, 52.

Office of Population Censuses and Surveys (1984) *Population Trends*, no. 36, London, HMSO, 62.

Okely, J. (1977) 'Gypsy women: models in conflict', in S. Ardener (ed.), *Perceiving Women*, New York, Halstead, 55–86.

Oldershaw, K.L. (1975) *Contraception, Abortion and Sterilization in General Practice*, London, Henry Kimpton Publishers.

Ortner, S.B. (1974) 'Is female to male as nature is to culture?', in M.Z. Rosaldo and L. Lamphere (eds), *Woman, Culture and Society*, Stanford, CA, Stanford University Press, 67–87.

Pankhurst, C. (1913) *Suffragette*, 8 August 1913, 737.

Parish, P.A., Stimson, G.V., Mapes, R. and Cleary, J. (1976) 'Prescribing in general practice', *Journal of the Royal College of General Practitioners*, Supplement no. 1, vol. 26.

Parish, T.N. (1935) *Journal of Obstetrics and Gynaecology of the British Empire*, vol. 42, 1107.

Parmar, P. (1982) 'Gender, race and class: Asian women in resistance', in Centre for Contemporary Cultural Studies (ed.), *The Empire Strikes Back: Race and Racism in 70s Britain*, London, Hutchinson.

Parsons, T. (1951) *The Social System*, Glencoe, Illinois, The Free Press.

Passmore, R. and Robson, J.S. (1968) *A Companion to Medical Studies*, Oxford, Blackwell.

Payling Wright, P. and Symmers, W. (1966) *Systematic Pathology*, London, Longmans.

Peel, J. and Potts, M. (1971) *Textbook of Contraceptive Practice* (reprinted), Cambridge, CUP.

Pfeffer, N. and Woollett, A. (1983) *The Experience of Infertility*, London, Virago.

Phillips, A. and Rakusen, J. (1979) *Our Bodies Ourselves*, Harmondsworth, Penguin Books.

Phillips, T.B.W. (1973) Letter to *British Medical Journal*, vol. 2, 782.

Polani, P.E. (1977) 'Who's for amniocentesis?' *Lancet*, vol. ii, 1099.

Polani, P.E., Alberman, E., Berry, A.C., Blunt, C. and Singer, J.D. (1976) 'Chromosome abnormalities and maternal age', *Lancet*, vol. ii, 516–517.

Pollock, M. (1966) *Family Planning: A Handbook for the Doctor*, London, Bailliere, Tindall and Cassell.

Pollock, S. (1984) 'Refusing to take women seriously: "side effects" and the politics of contraception', in R. Arditti *et al.* (eds), *Test-tube Women: What Future for Motherhood?*, London, Pandora Press, 138–152.

Pollock, S. (1985) *Women, Sexuality and Contraception*, London, Routledge and Kegan Paul.

Potts, M. (1971) Letter to *British Medical Journal*, vol. 3.

Pyke, M. (1952) Letter to *British Medical Journal*, vol. 1, 1028.

Rakusen, J. (1981) 'Depo-Provera: the extent of the problem. A case study in the politics of birth control', in H. Roberts (ed.), *Women, Health and Reproduction*, London, Routledge and Kegan Paul, 75–108.

Rakusen, J. (1982a) 'Feminism and the politics of health', *Medicine in Society*, vol. 8, no. 1, 17–25.

Rakusen, J. and Davidson, N. (1982b) *Out of our Hands – What Technology does to Pregnancy*, London, Crucible Pan Books.

Rakusen, J. (1984) 'In pursuit of the perfect baby', *Women's Reproductive Rights Information Centre, Newsletter*, May/June.

Ramaswamy, S. and Smith, T. (1976) *Practical Contraception*, London, Pitman Medical.

Reitz, R. (1981) *Menopause: a Positive Approach*, London, Unwin Paperbacks. (First published 1977 by the Chilton Book Company in the USA.)

Rhodes, P. (1975) 'Keeping well', in British Medical Association Booklet *You and Your Baby, Part 1, From Pregnancy to Birth*, London, A Family Doctor Publication, 43–46.

Rich, A. (1977a) 'The theft of childbirth', in C. Dreifus (ed.), *Seizing our Bodies: The Politics of Women's Health*, New York, Vintage, 146–163.

Rich, A. (1977b) *Of Woman Born: Motherhood as Experience and Institution*, London, Virago. (First published 1976 in the USA.)

Richards, M.P.M. (1975) 'Innovation in medical practice: obstetricians and the induction of labour in Britain', *Social Science and Medicine*, vol. 9, no. 11/12, 595–602.

Riley, D. (1981) 'Feminist thought and reproductive control: the state and the "right to choose"', in The Cambridge Women's Studies Group, *Women in Society: Interdisciplinary Essays*, London, Virago Press.

Riley, D. (1983) *War in the Nursery: Theories of the Child and Mother*, London, Virago.

Robbins, S.L. (1974) *Pathologic Basis of Disease*, Philadelphia, Saunders.
Roberts, C.J., Elder, G.H., Lawrence, K.M., Woodhead, J.S., Hibbard, B.M., Evans, K.T., Roberts, A., Robertson, I.B. and Hoole, M. (1983) 'The efficacy of a serum-screening service for neural tube defects: The South Wales experience', *Lancet*, vol. i, 1315–1318.
Roberts, H. (1979) 'Women, social class and IUD use', *Women's Studies International Quarterly*, vol. 2, no. 1, 49–56.
Roberts, H. (1981a) 'Male hegemony in family planning', in H. Roberts (ed.), *Women, Health and Reproduction*, London, Routledge and Kegan Paul, 1–17.
Roberts, H. (ed.) (1981b) *Women, Health and Reproduction*, London, Routledge and Kegan Paul.
Roberts, H. (1984) 'Begging for the needle and the knife', *Radical Community Medicine*, no. 17, Spring, 1–7.
Roberts, M.B.V. (1976) *Biology: A Functional Approach*, Sunbury-on-Thames, Nelson.
Robson, J. *et al.* (1977) *Quality, Inequality and Health Care. Notes on Medicine, Capital and the State.* A special edition of *Medicine in Society*, London, Marxists in Medicine, April.
Rogers, S.C., Weatherall, J.A.C. (1976) *Anencephalus, Spina Bifida and Congenital Hydrocephalus: England and Wales 1964–1972*, OPCS Studies on medical and population subjects, no. 32, London, HMSO.
Roggencamp, V. (1984) 'Abortion of a special kind: male sex selection in India', in R. Arditti *et al.* (eds), *Test-tube Women: What Future for Motherhood?*, London, Pandora Press, 266–277.
Ronalds, C., Vaughan, J.P. and Sprackling, P. (1977) 'Asian mothers' use of general-practitioner and maternal/child welfare services', *Journal of the Royal College of General Practitioners*, May, 281–284.
Rosaldo, M.Z. (1974) 'Woman, culture and society: a theoretical overview', in M.Z. Rosaldo and L. Lamphere (eds), *Woman, Culture and Society*, Stanford, CA, Stanford University Press, 17–42.
Rose, H. and Hanmer, J. (1979) 'Women's liberation, reproduction, and the technological fix', in D.L. Barker and S. Allen (eds), *Sexual Divisions and Society: Process and Change*, London, Tavistock, 199–223.
Rosengren, W.R. (1961–62) 'Social instability and attitudes toward pregnancy as a social role', *Social Problems*, vol. 9, 371–378.
Roszak, T. (1969) *The Making of a Counter-Culture: Reflections on the Technocratic Society and its Youthful Opposition*, Garden City, New York, Anchor Books.
Rowbotham, S. (1974) *Hidden from History: 300 Years of Women's Oppression and the Fight against it*, London, Pluto Press (2nd edn).
Rowland, R. (1984) 'Reproductive technologies: the final solution to the woman question', in R. Arditti *et al.* (eds), *Test-tube Women: What Future for Motherhood?*, London, Pandora Press, 356–369.
Royal Commission on the National Health Service (1979) *Report*, London, HMSO, Cmnd 7615.
Rush, F. (1981) *The Best Kept Secret: Sexual Abuse of Children*, New York, McGraw-Hill.
Russell, J. (1982) 'Perinatal mortality: the current debate', *Sociology of Health and Illness*, vol. 4, no. 3, 302–319.
Ruzek, S. (1979) *The Women's Health Movement*, New York, Praeger.
Ruzek, S. (1980) 'Medical response to women's health activities: conflict, accommodation and cooptation', *Research in the Sociology of Health Care*, vol. 1, 335–354.
Sadler, A. (1952a), Letter to *British Medical Journal*, vol. 1, 868.
Sadler, A. (1952b), Letter to *British Medical Journal*, vol. 1, 1132.

St George, D. (1983) 'The prevention of neural tube defects: a public health approach', *Nutrition and Health*, vol. 2, no. 2, 71–75.

Salisbury, G.W., Hart, R.G. and Lodge, J.R. (1976) 'The life of spermatozoa', *Biology and Medicine*, Winter 1976, 213–227.

Satow, A. and Homans, H. (1981) 'Integration or isolation?', *Journal of Community Nursing*, October, 4–5.

Savage, W. (1982) 'Taking liberties with women: abortion, sterilisation and contraception', *International Journal of Health Services*, vol. 12, no. 2, 293–308.

Saxton, M. (1984) 'Born and unborn: the implications of reproductive technologies for people with disabilities', in R. Arditti *et al.* (eds) *Test-tube Women: What Future for Motherhood?*, London, Pandora Press, 298–312.

Sayers, J. (1982) *Biological Politics*, London, Tavistock.

Scambler, A. and Versluysen, M. (1976) *Register of Research on Human Reproduction*, British Sociological Association, October.

Scazzocchio, C. (1982) 'The limits of biological reductionism', in S. Rose (ed.), *Towards a Liberatory Biology*, London, Allison and Busby, 79–84.

Schofield, M. (1976) *Promiscuity*, London, Victor Gollanz.

Schwartz, L.R. (1969) 'The hierarchy of resort in curative practices. The Admiralty Islands, Melanesia', *Journal of Health and Social Behaviour*, vol. 10, 201–209.

Scottish Home and Health Department (1981) *Scottish Health Bulletin*, Scotland, SHHD.

Scully, D. and Bart, P. (1978) 'A funny thing happened on the way to the orifice', in J. Ehrenreich (ed.), *The Cultural Crisis of Modern Medicine*, New York, Monthly Review Press, 212–226.

Seaman, B. and Seaman, G. (1978) *Women and the Crisis in Sex Hormones*, New York, Bantam Books.

Sedgwick, P. (1982) *Psychopolitics*, London, Pluto.

Seller, M.J. (1981) 'Maternal alpha-fetoprotein screening: 2 years' experience in a low-risk district', *British Medical Journal*, vol. 283, 1261–1262.

Short, R. (1979) 'Sexual selection and its component parts, somatic and genital-selection, as illustrated by man and the great apes', a review in *Advanced Study and Behaviour*, vol. 9, 131–158.

Simms, M. (1971) 'The Abortion Act after three years', *Political Quarterly*, vol. 42, no. 3, 269–287.

Simms, M. (1981) 'Abortion and the myth of the Golden Age', in B. Hutter and G. Williams (eds), *Controlling Women: The Normal and the Deviant*, London, Croom Helm, 168–184.

Simon, H. (1957) *Models of Man: Social and Rational*, New York, Wiley.

Simpson, K. (1949) *Lancet*, vol. 1, 47 and 48.

Sjoström, H. and Nilsson, R. (1972) *Thalidomide and the Power of the Drug Companies*, Harmondsworth, Penguin Books.

Smalley, C. and Bissenden, J. (1977) 'The Asian mother and baby at Sorrento', *The Journal of Maternal and Child Health*, October, 408–412.

Smith, D.J. (1980) *Overseas Doctors in the National Health Service*, London, Policy Studies Institute.

Smith, D.M. (1978) *General Urology*, Los Altos, California, Lange Medical Publications.

Social Services Committee on Perinatal and Neonatal Morality (1980) *Second Report*, House of Commons Paper 663–1 (Session 1979–80), London, HMSO.

Sontag, S. (1978) 'The double standard of ageing', in V. Carver and P. Liddiard (eds), *An Ageing Population*, Sevenoaks, Hodder and Stoughton, 72–80.

Special Article (1980) 'The morphology of spermatozoa – three centuries of microscopy', *British Journal of Sexual Medicine*, vol. 7, 12–22.

Spender, D. (1980) *Man Made Language*, London, Routledge and Kegan Paul.

Speroff, L., Glass, R.H. and Kase, N.G. (1979) *Clinical Gynaecologic endocrinology and infertility*, Baltimore, Williams and Wilkins.

Standing, J.S., Brindle, M.J., MacDonald, A.P. and Lacey, R.W. (1981) 'Maternal alpha-fetoprotein screening: 2 years' experience in a low-risk district', *British Medical Journal*, vol. 283, 705–707.

Stimson, G.V. (1976) 'Doctor–patient interaction and some problems for prescribing', in P.A. Parish *et al.* (eds), 'Prescribing in General Practice', *Journal of the Royal College of General Practitioners*, Supplement no. 1, vol. 26, 88–96.

Stimson, G.V. and Webb, B. (1975) *Going to see the Doctor: the Consultation Process in General Practice*, London, Routledge and Kegan Paul.

Stoller Shaw, N. (1974) *Forced Labour, Maternity Care in the United States*, Oxford, Pergamon Press.

Tietz, C. (1983) *Induced Abortion: a World Review*, New York, Population Council.

Torkington, P. (1983) *The Racial Politics of Health – a Liverpool Profile*, University of Liverpool, Department of Sociology.

Townsend, P. and Davidson, N. (1982) *Inequalities in Health*, Harmondsworth, Penguin Books.

Toynbee, P. (1981) 'The scandal is that so many handicapped babies are born at all', *Guardian*, 23 October, 12.

UK Collaborative Study on Alpha-fetoprotein in Relation to Neural Tube Defects (1977) 'Maternal serum-alpha-fetoprotein measurement in antenatal screening for anencephaly and spina bifida in early pregnancy', *Lancet*, vol. 1, 1323–1332.

Vaughan, P. (1972) *The Pill on Trial*, Harmondsworth, Penguin Books.

Waddy, S.H. (1952) Letter to *British Medical Journal*, vol. 1 867.

Waite, M. (1974) *Consultant Gynaecologists and Birth Control*, London, Birth Control Trust.

Wald, N., Cuckle, H.S. and Harwood, C.A. (1979) 'Screening for open neural tube defects in England and Wales', *British Medical Journal*, vol. 2, 331.

Walker, A. (1980) 'The social origins of impairment, disability and handicap', *Medicine in Society*, vol. 6, nos. 2 and 3, 18–26.

Walters, M. (1979) *The Male Nude*, Harmondsworth, Penguin Books.

Warnock Report (1984) *Report of the Committee of Inquiry into Human Fertilisation and Embryology*, London, HMSO.

Weare, T. (1979) 'Round in a flat world', *Spare Rib*, no. 78, January, 15–17.

Webb, C. and Wilson-Barnett, J. (1983) 'Coping with hysterectomy', *Journal of Advanced Nursing*, vol. 8, 311–319.

Weideger, P. (1978) *Female Cycles*, London, The Women's Press.

Weiss, K. (1975) 'What medical students learn about women', *Off our Backs*, April/May, 24–25.

White, L.A. (1959) *The Evolution of Culture*, New York, McGraw-Hill.

Whitten, N.E. and Whitten, D.S. (1972) 'Social strategies and social relationships', *Annual Review of Anthropology*, vol. 1, Palo Alto, CA, Annual Reviews Inc. 247–270.

Wilson, A. (1978) *Finding a Voice. Asian Women in Britain*, London, Virago.

Wilson, E. (1971) 'Domiciliary family planning in Glasgow', *British Medical Journal*, vol. 4, 731.

Wolf, M. (1972) *Women and the Family in Rural Taiwan*, Stanford, CA, Stanford University Press.

Woolf, M. (1971) *Family Intentions*, London, HMSO.

Young, R.M. (1979) 'Why are figures so significant? The role and critique of quantification', in J. Irvine *et al.* (eds), *Demystifying Social Statistics*, London, Pluto, 63–74.

Zola, I.K. (1979) 'Culture and symptoms. An analysis of patients' presenting complaints', in G.L. Albrecht and P.C. Higgins (eds) *Health, Illness and Medicine: a Reader in Medical Sociology*, Chicago, Rand McNally College Publishing Company, 41–62.

Useful Addresses

Abortion Law Reform Association
881 Islington High Street
LONDON N1

Association for Improvements in the Maternity Services (AIMS)
163 Liverpool Road
LONDON N1 0RF

Association for Spina Bifida and Hydrocephalus
22 Upper Woburn Place
LONDON WC1H 0EP

Black Health Workers and Patients Group
257–259 High Road
LONDON N15

British Pregnancy Advisory Service
Head Office
Austy Manor
Wootton Wawen
SOLIHULL
West Midlands

Brook Advisory Centre
153a East Street
LONDON SE17

Christians for a Free Choice
c/o V. Lukey
84 Colwith Road
LONDON W6

Co-ordinating Committee in Defence of the 1967 Abortion Act
(Co-ord)
27–35 Mortimer Street
LONDON W1

Down's Children Association
3rd Floor
4 Oxford Street
LONDON W1N 9FL

Feminist Self Insemination Group
Box 3
Sisterwrite
190 Upper Street
LONDON N1

International Contraception, Abortion and Sterilisation Campaign
52/54 Featherstone Street
LONDON EC1

Liberation Network for People with Disabilities
c/o 68 Alden House
Duncan Road
LONDON EC8

Marie Stopes House
108 Whitfield Street
LONDON W1T 6BE

The Miscarriage Association
Dolphin Cottage
4 Ashfield Terrace
Thorpe
WAKEFIELD
West Yorkshire

National Abortion Campaign (NAC)
75 Kingsway
LONDON WC2

Patients' Association
Room 33
18 Charing Cross Road
LONDON WC2H 0HR

Pregnancy Advisory Service
11/13 Charlotte Street
LONDON W1

Sisters Against Disablement
2 Mereworth Drive
Shooters Hill
LONDON SE3

Women in Medicine
12 Worple Avenue
LONDON SW19

Women's Health Group for Ethnic Minorities
c/o Aliyay Osman
8 Loveday Road
LONDON W13

Women's Health Information Centre (WHIC)
52/54 Featherstone Street
LONDON EC1

Women's Reproductive Rights Information Centre (WRRIC)
52/54 Featherstone Street
LONDON EC1

Name Index

Aitken-Swan, Jean 7, 45
Alberman, Eva 93, 98, 103
Allen, I. 93
Amelar, R.D. 38
Arditti, R. 11
Armstrong, David 35
Arthur, Leonard 95
Ashton, J.R. 93
Austin, C. 40

Baird, Dugald Sir 86
Baldwin, S. 99
Barker-Benfield, Ben 5
Barnes, J. 54–5, 57
Barrett, Michele 153
Bart, Pauline 32
Barth, F. 137
Beckett, S. 146
Begley, D.J. 40
Benson, R.C. 140
Berry, A.C. 103
Best, Sandy 5
Bissenden, Jeffrey 141
Beveridge (Report) 7
Birke, Linda 5
Birkett (Committee) 79–80
Bishop, W.M. 40
Black, Douglas Sir 100–1, 104, 110–12, 116
Bland, Lucy 7
Blum, R. 146
Bone, Margaret 45
Bourne, Aleck 80, 83
Bowlby, John 82
Boyson, Rhodes MP 105
Bradbury, Malcolm 59
Bradshaw, Jan 14
Braine, Bernard Sir 105
Brown, Judith 123
Browner, C. 126–7
Bruhn, J.A. 152
Bunge, R.G. 38
Burger, H. 37, 43

Campbell, Stuart 96
Carby, Hazel 3, 141
Carter, F.A. 100
Cartwright, Ann 92, 98, 141, 146, 150, 153
Chacko, Arun 10
Chalmers, Ian 104
Chamberlain, Mary 146
Chard, T. 100, 103
Chesser, E. 79
Chodorow, Nancy 124
Christopher, Elphis 8, 45
Conrad, P. 23
Corrie, John MP 105
Cossey, D. 58
Currie-Cohen, M. 130

Daly, Mary 5, 12, 17, 31
Davidson, Nick 9, 104
Davies, T.B. *et al.* 140

Davin, Anna 7
Davis, A. 92
Davis, Angela 3, 5
Day, Patricia 153
Day, Shelley 9, 99, 103
de Beauvoir, Simone 30–1, 44, 139
Dennis, K.J. 93
Deutsch, Helen 139
Dewhurst, J. 101
Doering, S.G. 129
Donald, Ian Professor 105
Donovan, Jenny 141, 151
Doyal, Lesley 5, 7–8, 66, 99–100, 103, 117, 153
Dubin, L. 38
Duelli Klein, Renate 2, 11
Dumont, T.L. 127
Dunnell, Karen 45, 92, 141, 146, 150

Edholm, Felicity 3, 124
Ehrenreich, Barbara 4–5, 31, 146
Elston, Mary Ann 31, 103, 117, 153, 160
English, Deirdre 5, 31, 146
Enkin, Murray 104
Entwistle, D.R. 129

Fabe, M. 131
Faithorn, E. 3
Farrant, Wendy 2, 3, 8–10, 109
Farrell, Christine 66
Fawcett, D. 33–4
Finch, Janet 99
Finegold, W. 129
Finger, Anne 10, 119
Fisher, S. 45
Flowers, Denise 28
Foster, G. 126
Frankl, G. 68
Freidson, Eliot 152
Freund, M. 41
Friberg, J. 38
Galtung, J. 42
Garcia, Jo 98
Garland, G.W. 153
Gemzell, C. 38
Gifford, P.W. 47, 50–1
Glass, N. 100
Glendinning, C. 99
Gordon, Linda 66–7
Goshen-Gottstein, E. 141
Graham, Hilary 6, 98–9, 103, 113, 137, 139, 143, 152
Grant, J.M. 5, 36
Gray, Judith 31
Greenwood, Victoria 66, 105
Groves, Dulcie 99
Guillebaud, John 59, 62

Hagard, S. 100
Haire, Doris 139
Hampson, Keith MP 96, 101, 105, 119
Hanmer, Jalna 10, 11
Harris, C.M. 152
Harrison, N. 39
Hearn, K. 121
Helman, Cecil 152, 155
Hern, Warren M. 141
Herschberger, Ruth 34–5, 38, 40, 42–3
Herxheimer, A. 141, 146
Hindell, Keith 66, 78
Hite, Shere 25–6
Hoffman, L.W. 129
Holmes, Helen B. 10
Holterman, S. 100
Homans, Hilary 2, 3, 6, 9–10, 12, 99, 141, 145–6, 149, 152–4
Hooks, Bell 3
Hornstein, Francie 11
Hoskins, Betty B. 10
Hubbard, Ruth 32
Hudson, B. 37, 42–3
Humphreys, Charlotte 104
Hunter, N.D. 132

Hussein, I.Y. 5, 36

Jackson, Stevi 66–7
Jeffrey, Patricia 10
Jeffrey, Roger 10
Jones, B.F.S. 49

Kaplan, A. 41
Kitzinger, Sheila 3
Klass, Alan 156
Kreitman, K. 146

Lane, Elizabeth Justice 89–90, 93
Langford, C.M. 45
Larned, D. 5
Law, B. 57
Laws, Sophie 2–4, 12, 16, 28, 70
Leathard, Audrey 45, 66
Ledward, R.S. 130
Leeson, Joyce 31
Leeuwenhoek, Antoni van 39, 42
Lennane, K. 15, 140
Lennane, R.J. 15, 140
Lever, Judy 13
Lewin, Ellen 2–3, 11–12, 126–7, 132
Lewis, Jane 7, 66, 103
Lewis, T.L.T. 85
Lindenbaum, S. 3
Lipshultz, L.T. 38
Littlefield, J.W. 119
Luttrell, L. 130

MacFarlane-Burnett, I.B. 39
Macintyre, Sally 1, 6, 45, 50, 63
Mackay, E. 51
MacKeith, Nancy 12, 45
Macnicol, John 7
Malleson, Jean 48
Mann, T. 41
Marieskind, Helen 5, 30
Mason, Micheline 99, 119, 121
Mass, Bonnie 5
Meredith, P. 58
Merrison (Committee) 94–5
Minden, Shelley 11
Mitchell, Jeanette 140, 150
Moench, Conrad 41
Mozans, H.T. 37

Nelson, C.M.K. 38
Nichter, Mark 145
Nicolas, P. 47, 49
Nicolas, S. 47, 49
Nilsson, Robert 158
Norbeck, Edward 22
Notley, R. 36

Oakley, Ann 1, 6, 31, 98, 113, 139, 152
O'Brien, Mary 4
Okely, Judith 3
Oldershaw, K.L. 49, 53, 56–60
Ortner, Sherry 124

Pankhurst, Christabel 6
Parish, T.N. 92
Parmar, Pratibha 141
Parsons, O.A. 152
Parsons, Talcott 141
Passmore, R. 33, 39, 42
Payling Wright, P. 33, 41
Peel, J. 53, 55
Pfeffer, Naomi 2, 3, 5, 12, 36
Phillips, Angela 12, 45, 146
Phillips, T.B.W. 53
Polani, P.E. 98
Polikoff, N.D. 132
Pollock, M. 52, 60
Pollock, Scarlet 2, 4–5
Potts, Malcolm 51, 53, 55
Pyke, Margaret 47, 49

Rakusen, Jill 8–9, 12, 45, 52, 65, 98–9, 121, 146
Ramaswamy, S. 46, 55–6, 59, 61–2

Reeves, Joseph MP 80
Reitz, Rosetta 5, 146
Rhodes, Professor 153
Rich, Adrienne 4–5, 13, 31, 139
Richards, M.P.M. 100, 103
Richardson, Jo MP 95
Riley, Denise 2, 105
Robbins, S.L. 34–5
Roberts, C.J. 104
Roberts, Helen 65–6, 103, 117, 153
Roberts, M.B.V. 36
Robinson, Kenneth MP 81
Robson, John 153
Robson, J.S. 33, 39, 42
Roche, Sheila 1
Rogers, S.C. 109
Roggencamp, Viola 10
Ronalds, Claire 141
Rosaldo, Michelle Zimbalist 124
Rose, Hilary 11
Rosengren, William R. 141
Roszak, Theodore 138
Rowbotham, Sheila 7
Rowland, Robyn 9–10
Rush, Florence 29
Russell, Jill 103
Ruzek, Sheryl 30, 137

Sadler, A. 47–9
St George, David 104
Salisbury, G.W. 37
Satow, Antoinette 141, 153
Savage, Wendy 8
Saxton, Marsha 10, 119
Sayers, Janet 2, 31
Scambler, Annette 1
Scazzochio, C. 42
Schofield, Michael 66
Schwartz, Lola R. 146
Scott, J.S. 101
Scully, Diana 32
Seaman, Barbara 65, 146
Seaman, Gideon 65, 146
Sedgwick, Peter 31
Seller, M.J. 104
Shapiro, S. 130
Short, R. 37
Short, Renee MP 81
Silkin, Lord 81–2
Simms, Madeleine 2, 7–8, 66, 78, 92, 94
Simpson, K. 92
Sjostrom, Henning 158
Smalley, Christine 141
Smith, David J. 153
Smith, D.M. 35, 42
Smith, T. 46, 55–6, 59, 61–2
Sontag, Susan 43
Spender, Dale 32
Speroff, L. 34
Standing, J.S. 104
Steel, David MP 81–2
Steinem, Gloria 23
Stimson, Gerry 141, 146, 151, 156
Stoller Shaw, Nancy 6, 139
Symmers, W. 33, 41

Thomas, Hilary 2, 4–5, 9
Thurtle, Dorothy 80
Tietz, Christopher 85, 87
Torkington, Protasia 141
Townsend, Peter 104
Toynbee, Polly 96

Vaughan, P. 65
Versluysen, Margaret 1

Waddy, S.M. 49
Waite, M. 106
Wald, N. 98
Walker, Alan 104
Walters, Margaret 37
Walton, A. 40
Warnock (Committee Report) 9
Weare, Tessa 139
Weatherall, J.A.C. 109
Webb, Christine 5

Weideger, Paula 14
Weiss, Kay 5
White, Leslie 22, 28
Whitten, D.S. 125
Whitten, N.E. 125
Wikler, N. 131
Wilson, Amrit 140–1, 150
Wilson, Elizabeth 47, 51
Wilson-Barnett, Jenifer 5
Wingfield Digby, Simon MP 81
Wolf, Margery 127
Woolf, M. 45
Woollett, Anne 2, 36

Young, Jock 66, 105
Young, R.M. 38

Zola, Irving 140

Subject Index

abortion 6
  and amniocentesis 10, 96, 103, 105–8, 118
  and contraception 47, 50–1, 57
  and foetal abnormality 89, 96, 106–18
  and Parliamentary activity 80–3, 90–1, 95
  and prenatal screening 96, 103, 110, 113–17, 119
  and women's groups 91, 95
  charities 86–7, 90
  confidentiality of 94
  counselling 87, 91, 116
  death from 8, 79, 87–90
  illegal 79–80, 85, 92, 95
  legislation 2, 7, 47, 50, 79–95, 105
  numbers of 47, 84–6, 92–4
  opponents of 95, 106
  private 79, 85–7, 94
  provision 8, 66, 78, 84–7, 93–4
  regional inequalities 8, 86–7, 93–4
  right to choose 10, 94, 105
  safety of 80, 92
  septic 87, 91–2
  spontaneous 107
  social grounds for 84, 86, 94, 106
  time of 87, 89–90, 93, 95
  waiting lists for 93
Abortion Act 1967 8, 47, 50, 78, 83–7, 89–94
Abortion Law Reform Association 78, 81–2, 86, 91–2
'acculturation' 146
Adam's Rib 34
adultery and artificial insemination 130
ageing 35, 43
allopathy 146, 150
  see also medicine
alphafetoprotein (AFP) 97–8, 101–4, 109–12, 115–17, 121
  national programme of screening for 102
  regional programme of screening for 109–10
amniocentesis 9–10, 121, 137
  and age of women 111, 113
  and foetal abnormality 10
  and sex determination 10
  costs of 103–4
  counselling 10, 97, 109–13, 116–17, 119
  hazards of 10, 104, 111–13
  policy of 97
  women's choice 111–13
    see also prenatal screening

antenatal care 6, 98, 100–1, 110, 113, 138
individualised 161
women challenging 161
antenatal clinic 140, 154
antenatal intervention 98–9, 100–1, 139, 161
anthropologists 3
cultural 137
feminist 123
Marxist 124
antropology
of gender 123–5, 136–7
anthropometrics 37
anti abortionists 78, 81–2, 86, 90–1, 95, 97, 105, 120
artificial insemination 2, 38, 129–36
and adultery 130
and autonomy 129, 136
anonymity of donor 129, 132–6
by donor (AID) 9, 11, 130–6
Association for Improvements in the Maternity Services (AIMS) 102
Ayurveda 145, 149

Bhandari clinic (Amritsar, India) 10
Bibliography on the Sociology of Human Reproduction 1
biological theories 30
constraints 124
determinism 2
perspectives 124
biology
functional 36
male 38
textbooks 36, 41
birth control 66, 78, 83
campaigners for 7, 66
clinics 6
see also contraception, family planning, fertility control
Birth Control Trust 45
birth rate 79
black culture 3
history 141
people 140–1, 153, 161
women 3, 5, 8, 12, 113
and sterilisation 8
see also ethnic minority groups
Black Report on AFP screening 100–2, 110–12, 116
blood 150
'bad' 149
'bloodlessness' 149
high blood pressure 149–50
tests 121, 154
see also menstruation
British Medical Association (BMA) 79, 153
British Medical Journal (BMJ) 45–8, 50–2, 60–1, 96, 99
British Pregnancy Advisory Service (BPAS) 8, 11, 86–8
British Sociological Association (BSA) 1
Brook Advisory Centres 83

cancer
of prostrate 35
Capital Radio 28
cervical cap 45
see also contraception
cervix 32, 39
chemist *see* pharmacist
chemist's shop 150–2
Chief Medical Officer 78–9, 84
childbearing 61, 63, 124
elderly 63, 137
risks of 62, 80, 87–8, 98
childbirth 2, 31, 36, 137
first 63
childrearing 123–4
children 127–9
adoption of 131
and loyalty 126
custody of 131–2, 135

children (cont.)
  desire for 131
  meaning of 126
China
  sex predetermination in 10
Chinese women 127
Christians for Free Choice 91
Church, the 80
  and domination of women 67
  of England and abortion 80, 91
  Roman Catholic 81, 83, 85–6, 90–1, 120
Clinical Genetics Society 98, 101–3, 120
coil *see* intra uterine contraceptive device (IUCD)
communication
  cultural variations 153
  doctor–patient 153
Community Health Council (CHC) News 96
conception 32, 37–43
Conservative Party, the 81
consumer interest 87, 99
  organisations 96
contraception 1, 5, 45–77
  access to 45, 51
  and men 45, 53–4
  and menstrual blood 70
  and pharmacists 58
  and sex 67–77
  cost of 51
  female methods of 45, 53–4, 58–60, 71–4
  functions of 46–50
  male methods of 53–4, 58, 60, 64, 73, 75–6
  non-mechanical means of 42, 45
  social factors affecting 46–63
  struggle for 7, 66
  see also birth control
contraceptive 'career' 5, 45–63
  choice 1, 52–60, 62–3
  design 64
  development 64, 67
  facilities 66, 92
  methods 4, 8–9, 45–77
  needs 46, 60–2
  technology 4, 64–5, 76
  use 64, 67
contraceptives
  and breast feeding 54, 62
  and contra-indications 52, 55
  and female control over 73–6
  effectiveness of 55–6, 61–2, 64–5, 72–7
  motivation to use 53, 56–8
  side effects of 47, 62, 65, 71–2, 75–6
  suitability of 46, 52, 61
  variety of 46, 61
Co-ordinating Committee in Defence of the 1967 Abortion Act (Co-ord) 91
cultural behaviour 137
  constraints 126
  construction of gender 123, 136–7
  diversity 123–4
  factors 8
  ideas 13
  norms 45
  practices 2–3
    and contraception 58, 68
culture
  American 127–8
  'exotic' 146
  female 3–4
  male 2–4, 12, 12–29
  sexist 15–16
  white 3, 13–14, 68
  youth 138
cystitis 31, 143

Daily Express 96
Daily Mail 81
Debendox 158

decision making
and abortion 113–17
and amniocentesis 110–13
and motherhood 11, 123–38
and Parliament 7
Department of Health and Social Security (DHSS) 89, 99–101, 104, 110, 112, 116
Depo Provera (DP) 44, 57, 65
and black and Asian women 8
see also contraception
desi 146, 150
see also home cures
diaphragm 45, 47, 53, 57, 59, 62, 70–3
see also contraception
diet
and health maintenance 145–50, 155, 157, 160
'balanced' 145–7
see also food, nutrition
Director of Public Prosecutions (DPP) 95
digestive disorders in pregnancy 139–40, 143–5, 147–8, 151, 153, 155–8
disabilities 9, 97, 99, 117, 119–21
babies with 9, 96, 99, 114–18
prevention of 99–100, 103–5, 107–8, 118
discomforts in pregnancy 139–61
and drugs 150–9
and mobility 143, 154
and work 143–5
GPs reaction to 152–9
incidence of 140
normality of 152–3, 160
see also illness, minor
Distaval 158
see also drugs in pregnancy
doctor–patient interaction 152–3, 159
doctors 4, 10, 30, 34, 89, 96, 140, 153, 155
and amniocentesis 96
and artificial insemination 130–2, 135–6
and curing 152–3, 156–8
and family planning 44, 47, 49, 51–2, 61–3
and folk beliefs 152, 160
and social background 153
dependency on 160–1
hospital 152
male 4, 153
see also general practitioners, medical profession
domestic sphere 124
Down's syndrome 98, 100, 103, 108–9, 114–15
drug companies
and contraception 67
and prenatal screening 102–3
drug therapy for reproductive disorders 35
drugs
in pregnancy 150–61
self medication 141, 146, 150–2
side effects of 47, 55, 62, 71–2, 75–6, 158–61
see also medical prescriptions
dysmenhorrhea 31

Edinburgh Sunday Standard 86
embryo transfer 11
ethnic minority groups
health needs of 140, 153, 161
women 5, 8–9, 89, 97
ethnicity 137
etiquette 4, 22, 28–9
and male culture 27–9
menstrual 22–4
within heterosexual relationship 24–7
eugenics 105, 107–8, 119
euthanasia 108

Evening News 11
exercise and health maintenance 145

fallopian tubes 32
family 65, 126, 129, 132
  Catholic 133
  conventional 128
  patriarchal 65–6
  ties 129
  uterine 127
Family Endowment Society 7
family planning 46–50, 52, 54–6, 58, 61–2, 65–7
  clinics 6, 48, 58
  doctors 44, 47, 49, 51–2, 61–3
  domiciliary 51
  international 66
  programmes 65–6
  services 45, 63
  see also birth control, contraception
Family Planning Association (FPA) 48
father, biological 43, 129, 134–5
fatherhood 43, 124
female contraception *see* contraception
female experiences 12, 16, 139
Female Trouble 29
femininity 70–1, 126–7, 140
feminism, modern 82–3
feminist anthropologists 123
  analyses 3, 12, 13–15, 29, 31, 38, 43–4
  critique of medicine 31–2
  issues 64
  literature 5, 12, 45
  politics 11, 134
feminists
  and abortion 82–3, 90
  anti 91
  black 3
  radical 3–4
  white 3
Feminist Self Insemination Group (London) 11
fertilisation *see* conception
fertility
  control over 3, 6–7, 11, 45, 92
  female 36–8, 54, 63, 65
  language of 32
  male 5, 40–3
  measures of 32, 36–43
  period of 133
Fertility and Sterility 38
foetal abnormality 9–10, 62, 79, 81
  and abortion 89, 96, 105–8, 113–17, 120
  and drugs in pregnancy 81, 158
  and prenatal diagnosis 96–121
folk beliefs about health and illness 140, 146, 150, 152, 160–1
  and doctors 152, 155
  undermining of 161
folk medicine 146–50, 152, 155, 161
  see also traditional recipes
food
  avoidance of during pregnancy 145, 147
  'cold' 145, 147
  fatty 147–8
  home cures 146–50, 155
  'hot' 145, 147
  production and processing of 104
  prohibition of, during pregnancy 145–6
  see also diet, nutrition
Freethinkers 78
friends and health care 145
  see also lay support system

functionalists 141

gender 38, 44
  anthropology of 123, 136
genetic counselling 102
geneticists 98, 101–3, 120
general practitioners 6, 11, 45–6, 53, 57–8, 61, 140
  and abortion 83, 93
  and antenatal care 139, 152
  and lay beliefs 152, 160
  and pregnancy discomforts 153–6
  and prescribing in pregnancy 156–61
  see also doctors
goals, achieved 125–7, 137
government
  and abortion 79–84, 89–91, 94–5
  and prenatal screening 99–100
  and sanitary wear 28
  Conservative 89
  Labour 82–3
Greenham Common 23
Guardian, the 96, 101, 119, 158
Gujerat (India) 161
gynaecological care 30
gynaecologists 15, 34, 45, 50, 80, 86, 93, 101, 117
gynaecology 3, 32–4, 96

handicap *see* disabilities
healing
  and women 145–6, 150, 160–1
health administrators
  and abortion 89
health authorities
  area 97, 98
  district 121
  regional 100, 102, 109–10
health
  and social policies 99
  care systems 122, 129, 133, 137
  maintenance 145–6, 160–1
  restoration 146–161
  social factors affecting 143–5
Heavy Periods 29
Hells Angels 29
hierarchy of resort 146
home cures 141, 146–50, 155, 160–1
  see also desi, folk medicines, traditional recipes
homosexuals, male 134
  see also lesbian women
hormones 42
  female reproductive 34–5, 37
  male reproductive 34–5, 43
  replacement therapy 35
hospitalisation 159
House of Commons 81, 83, 94, 100, 105
House of Lords 82, 84, 90
Human Reproduction Study Group 1, 2
husbands 113, 115, 144
hysterectomy 5, 36

iatrogenesis 100, 103
ideological interests 97
ideology 15–17, 119, 125, 127
  and medical practice 100, 104, 117
  medical 15, 103, 156
  see also patriarchal ideology
illegitimacy 47, 50–1, 66, 130–1
illness
  minor 6, 139–40, 142–61
  psychogenic 140, 160
  psychosomatic 15
  social definitions of 143–5
impotence 36, 43, 68
incest 29

India 140, 145–6
  sex predetermination in 10
Indian medical knowledge (traditional) *see* Ayurveda
individualism 125–9, 137
inequalities 8–9
  in abortion provision 86–7, 93–4
  see also National Health Service
infertility 2, 129–30
  female 39
  male 34, 38, 42–3, 129
International Planned Parenthood Federation (IPPF) 46, 52, 59, 61
intra uterine contraceptive device (IUCD) 8, 45, 47, 53–5, 57–8, 60–3, 64–5, 70–3, 75
  see also contraception
in vitro fertilisation (IVF) 9, 11, 40
  see also reproductive technology

Kenya 161
kin and health care 145–50, 160–1
kinship ties 124, 126–7, 137

Labour Party, the 78, 91, 94
  MPs 80–3, 95
language
  and pregnancy 139
  and reproductive medicine 5, 32–4, 38
  Asian 162
  English 145, 162
  sexism in 5, 17, 32, 36, 43–4, 67, 70
Latin American migrants 126–7
lawyers and abortion 89
lay support system 146, 160–1
legitimacy and artificial insemination 130
lesbians 11, 127–36
  and child custody 131–2, 135
  and counter culture 134
Liberal Party, the 81, 90
Liberation Network for People with Disabilities 119
Life 91, 95
liver, the 36
Lord Chief Justice 84

male
  contraceptives 53–4, 58, 60, 64, 73, 75–6
  control and reproduction 2–4, 6, 9, 11, 66–7, 130
    see also patriarchy
  culture 2–4, 12, 13–29
  doctors 4, 153
  fertility 5, 40–3
  impotence 36, 43, 68
  scientists 4, 9, 11
  sexual pleasure 4, 64, 67–73, 76–7
  virility 67–8, 76
Male Nude, The 37
marriage 47, 49–52, 61–2, 66, 83, 127, 139
masculinity 70, 126
masturbation 69, 130
maternal health services 140
  cuts in 101
  see also ante natal care
maternity and family allowances 7
Maternity Alliance 121
media and prenatal screening 96–7, 105, 118–19
medical
  journals/textbooks 4–5, 9, 32–3, 38, 45–63, 140, 153

medical (cont.)
  knowledge 2, 6, 32–44, 45–63
  prescriptions 152–61 *see also* drugs
  profession 2, 4–6, 9–11, 45–63, 66–7, 79, 83–4, 86, 89–91, 94–5, 97–9, 100–2, 111, 140, 152–61
  students 32
  supply industry 99, 102–3
Medical Research Council (MRC) 104, 111
Medical Women's Federation 47, 48
medicine and social control 15, 31, 36, 43–4, 63, 97
medicines *see* drugs
Members of Parliament (MPs) 80–1
  Catholic 81–2, 90–1, 105
  Conservative 81–2, 90, 96, 105
  Labour 80–1, 83, 90–1, 95, 105
  Liberal 81–2, 90
  women 95
men 14–29
  and contraception *see* contraception, male methods of
  as patients 30
  elderly 35–6
  fertility in 5, 40–3
  sexual liaisons with 131
  white 3, 14
menopause 31, 35, 42, 46
menstrual cycles 11, 16, 20, 32, 54
  blood 25–6, 70
  disorders 15
  etiquette 12, 13–29
  jokes 15, 18–21
  pain 2, 16
  taboo 4, 13, 29
menstruating women 23–7
menstruation 2, 4, 13–29, 31, 36
  and heterosexual relationships 16, 24
  and mood change 20, 23
  and mothers 24
  and pornography 19, 21, 70
  and sisters 24
  beliefs about 13–14
  'excessive' 5, 36
  hiding 16, 27, 29
  sexualisation of 27
midwives 45, 63, 100, 153, 155, Italian 80
migration 150, 161
Minister of Health 81
miscarriage 32, 104, 111–12, 118
morality and contraception 53, 66
'morning after' contraception 87 *see also* contraception
mother
  and health advice 146–7, 149
  death of 144, 155
motherhood
  AID 130–7
  and Latin American women 126–7
  and rational behaviour 11, 125
  as a resource 125, 136
  desire for 125–9, 131
  in patriarchal society 11, 140
  in state interventions 7
  lesbian 127–37
  single 130–7
  universal 15
mother-in-law 146, 149, 155
mothers
  and menstruation 15–16, 24
  as carers 99, 117
  Asian 140
  'at risk' 97

mothers (cont.)
  becoming and being 123, 129, 137, 139
  influence over daughters 15–16, 24
  physical and mental health of 80, 83
  unmarried 47, 49, 66, 134
  white 140
  women's role as 32, 49, 123–9
  working 82
mortality
  from abortion 8, 79, 87–90
  from tuberculosis 78
  infant 78
  maternal 78–9, 87–8
National Abortion Campaign (NAC) 91
National Health Service (NHS) 8, 50–1, 82, 92, 150
  abortions 84, 93–5, 106
  hospitals 84–7, 139
  inequalities in provision 8, 86–7, 93–5, 109–10
  prenatal screening 100, 102
  reorganisation 47, 98
  see also health administrators, health authorities
National Medical Consultative Committee 103
National Opinion Polls (NOP) 83, 94
nausea (vomiting) in pregnancy 139–40, 143–5, 147, 156–7
neural tube defects *see* spina bifida
North East Thames Regional Health Authority 109–10
nurses 44, 63, 153
  and abortion 90, 95
nutrition 104, 141, 145–6 *see also* diet, food

obstetricians 6, 93, 97–8, 100–1, 103, 106–8, 110–14, 119–20, 152
obstetrics 96, 99–101, 103
  history 98, 109
  textbook 153
Offences against the Persons Act 1861 79
Office of Population and Census Surveys (OPCS) 35, 85–6, 89
old wives' tales 36, 146, 160
oral contraception
  female 45, 47, 53–7, 59–63, 64–5, 70–5, 83
  male 75
  see also contraception
Outrageous Acts and Everyday Rebellions 23
over population 47, 51–2 *see also* population control
ovulation 32, 54, 133
ovum 32, 37, 39–41

Pakistan 161
palpitations 153 *see also* discomforts
parity 49, 80, 139, 143
paternity 124 *see also* fatherhood
patriarchal
  family life 65–6
  ideology 2, 14–29, 38, 67–77
  sexual relations 64–77
  social relations 2, 4, 12, 15, 29
penis 30, 33
perinatal medicine 96
  mortality and morbidity 100, 104
pessaries 59 *see also* contraception
pharmaceutical companies *see* drug companies
pharmacist 140–1, 150–2

pill, the *see* oral contraception
police, the
  and abortion 80, 91
politics
  and abortion 78–95
  of prenatal screening 96–122
  sexual 2, 13–29, 64–77
Pope, the 80
population control 7, 49, 51–2, 65–7
pornography 19, 21, 68, 70
post-natal depression 9
power
  and sex 67–9
  male 2, 13–29
Practical Conception 46
premenstrual tension (PMT) 13, 16, 20–1, 31
PMT 29
pregnancy 1, 8, 11, 13, 36, 86–8, 94, 99–100, 117, 139–61
  and age 66, 103, 109, 139
  and health 2, 47, 62, 139, 140–6, 160–1
  and lesbian women 127–37
  as 'natural' 6, 139, 152, 160
  as pathological 6, 139, 152, 160
  drugs in 150–61
  ectopic 32
  hospitalisation during 159
  illness in 140–61
  images of 139 152–3, 160
  length of 108, 121, 154
  medical management of 99–100, 103, 137, 139
  preventing 47, 53, 55–6, 61–2, 66 *see also* contraception
  teenage 66
  termination of 113–17 *see also* abortion
  undesirable 47, 50
  unplanned 50, 61, 70
  unwanted 47–8, 50–3, 94, 107
Pregnancy Advisory Service (PAS) 8, 11, 86–7
pregnant women 99–100, 109–21
prenatal femicide 10
prenatal screening
  and consultants 103, 105–8, 112–14, 119–20
  costs of 103–4, 109–10, 118
  development of 97–103
  inequality in provision of 8, 109–10
  programmes 2, 8–9, 105–6
  vested interest in 99–103, 108–17
  women's experiences of 109–18
  women's right to 96, 120–1
  see also amniocentesis
Prevention and Health : Everybody's Business (1976) 100
Priorities for Health and Social Services in England (1976) 101
prostrate 33–6
psychiatrists 89, 94
psychosexual disorders 36, 46
public health 78
  sphere 124–5

quantitative analysis 38

race 8, 134, 153, 161
racism 3, 5–6, 8, 12, 14, 18, 66, 140–1, 161
rape 3, 68, 79–80
Red Rag 29
Reducing the Risk : Safer Pregnancy and Childbirth (1977) 99
Regional Genetic Advisory Centres 102
religion 137
  and abortion 6, 8, 79–83, 86, 90, 92–3, 119–20

religion (cont.)
  and AID 130
  and contraceptive use 8
religious pressure groups
  and abortion 78, 83, 91, 94–5
Report on the Medical Aspects of Abortion (1936) 79
Report of the Royal Commission on the National Health Service (1979) (Merrison Committee) 100
Report (Second) from the Social Services Committee on Perinatal and Neonatal Mortality (1980) 100
Report of Working Party of the Clinical Genetics Society (1978) 98–103
reproduction 1
  control over 2–6, 11–12, 52, 65, 105, 108, 113, 117, 120–1, 130
  knowledge of 2
  'normal' 6, 31
  planned 7
  politics of 1–2, 11, 13–29, 64–77, 78–95, 96–122
reproductive
  health 43–4
  organs 1, 4–5, 30, 37, 40, 43
  pathologies 1, 3, 5, 30–44
  strategies 123–38
  systems 2–3, 12, 30, 33–6
  technology 1–2, 9–11, 64–5, 94, 96–121, 130, 137
research 3, 8, 12, 17, 29, 65
rhythm method of contraception 43, 45, 72 *see also* contraception
Royal College of Obstetricians and Gynaecologists (RCOG) 101
'safe' period 47, 73 *see also* contraception
sanitary wear 16, 18–20
  public discussion of 16, 23–4, 27–9
  taxation of 16, 27–8
Scotland
  abortions in 79, 84–6
  prenatal screening in 109
Scottish Home and Health Department (SHHD) 84
Second Sex, The 30
Secretary of State 105
self insemination 11, 130–1, 133–6 *see also* artificial insemination
semen 33, 37–8, 42
sex 64–77, 153
  education 66
  predetermination 9–10
  roles 124
sexual
  assault *see* rape
  attractiveness 69–71
  availability 4, 59, 64, 74
  behaviour 1, 58–60, 71–3
  division of labour 123–4
  double standard 64, 67
  foreplay 69
  insults 15, 18–21, 27–9, 68
  intercourse 16, 24–7, 29, 51, 58–61, 64–5, 67–77
  liberation 4, 7, 64–5, 82
  medicine 52
  orgasm 68–9
  politics 1–2, 4, 11–12, 15, 27–9, 64–77, 78
  problems 60
  promiscuity 55, 66–7
  relations 4, 17, 58–60, 64–77
  responsibility 73–6
  spontaneity 58–60, 67–8

sexual (cont.)
surgery 5, 35–6
sexuality 1, 3, 67
black women's 3
heterosexual 2, 4, 9, 11, 15–17, 24–7, 54, 58–61, 64, 67–77, 127–8, 131 *see also* homosexuals, lesbian women
sexually transmitted disease 1, 6, 28, 46
sheaths (male contraceptives) 53–4, 58–60, 64, 71–3, 75 *see also* contraception
sick role 141–2
slavery 3
sleeplessness 142, 155, 159 *see also* discomforts
social
class 66, 89, 97, 139, 153, 158, 160–2
construction 2, 31, 43
factors 143–5
workers 89, 91, 94
Society for the Protection of the Unborn Child (SPUC) 91
South America, sterilisation in 5
Soviet Union, abortion in 80
sperm 33–4, 39–42, 129–33
spermatogenesis 31, 43
spermatozoa 33, 39–42
sperm banks 130
spermicides 47, 58–9, 71–3 *see also* contraception
spina bifida 96, 108
Standing Committee on Genetic Services 102
Standing Medical Advisory Group 100
state, the 2, 6–8, 67
sterilisation 5, 8, 55, 57, 62–3, 66, 76
sterility *see* infertility
stillbirth 104
Stopes, Marie clinic 8
strategy 125–6
stress and ill health 144
Student Health Service (Sheffield) 51
surgical operations 93 *see also* abortion, sterilisation, vasectomy
Systemic Pathology 33

taboos 3, 13–14, 22, 25, 29
tampons 16, 19, 23–4, 70 *see also* sanitary wear
Tanzania 161
teachers 83, 89, 145
termination of pregnancy *see* abortion
testicles 32–4, 37, 43
testis, cancer of 35
thalassaemia, screening for 109
thalidomide 81, 158 *see also* drugs in pregnancy
Times, The 28, 101
trade unions and abortion 91
traditional remedies 146–50, 155, 160–1 *see also* folk medicine

ultra-sound 101–3, 105, 110
United Kingdom Collaborative Study 98, 100
United States 5, 11, 119, 126–37
urinary system 34
urologists 30, 34–6, 38
uterus 32, 34, 39–40

vaginal infections 31, 143, 159
vaginal sponge 58 *see also* contraception
varicose veins 34, 144
vasectomy 38, 54, 76
venereal disease *see* sexually transmitted disease

Wales
prenatal screening in 109
withdrawal method of contraception 64, 71–3 *see also* contraception
women
abortion campaigners 78, 82–3, 91 *see also* abortion
and children 63, 126–9, 132–6, 144
and disability 12, 121
and nature 124, 138
and prenatal screening 109–18
and production 124
and risk of foetal abnormality 97–8, 108–10, 117, 120
as carers 99, 117, 137
as mothers 32, 49, 123–9
as patients 31, 43, 140, 150
as wives 32
Asian 8–9, 89, 140–1
black 3, 5, 8, 12, 89, 113, 141
Catholic 84–6, 133
Chinese 127
ethnic minority 8–9, 57–8, 97
'feckless' 49–50, 57
French 85
German 85
graduates 82
healing 145–6, 150, 160–1
Irish 85
Italian 85
Latin American 126–7
married 47, 49–52, 61–2, 66, 83, 127, 139
middle class 68, 79, 138, 158, 160–1
older 35, 140, 145–6, 160–1
Punjabi 9, 140–62
Spanish 85
white 3, 68, 140–61
wise 146
working 82, 92, 123–4, 131, 143–5
working class 12, 79, 89, 113, 146, 160, 162
young 66, 89
women's
advocates 106
health 43–4, 47, 62, 65, 71–2, 75–6, 79–80, 137, 139, 141–6, 160–1
status 13, 123–4
suffrage 78
Women's Liberation Movement, the 82–3, 91, 94
world wars
first 79
second 80, 82

You and Your Baby 145, 153